REVERSE TYPE 2 DIABETES FAST

A Proven Path to Lasting Health

RAJENDER KUMAR

Rajender Kumar

✲

Trademarks

Screenshots

Website References

Published by:
Jamba Academy

Printed in the United States of America

First Printing Edition, 2025

Found Typos & Broken Link

We apologize in advance for any typos or broken link that you may find in this book. We take pride in the quality of our content and strive to provide accurate and useful information to our readers. Please let us know where you found the typos and broken link (if any) so that we can fix them as soon as possible. Again, thank you very much in advance for bringing this to our attention and for your patience.

If you find any typos or broken links in this book, please feel free to email me.

support@JambaAcademy.com

Support

We would love to hear your thoughts and feedback! Could you please take a moment to write a review or share your thoughts on the book? Your feedback helps other readers discover the books and helps authors to improve their work. Thank you for your time and for sharing your thoughts with us!

If there is anything you want to discuss or you have a question about any topic of the book, you can always reach out to me, and I will try to help as much as I can.

support@JambaAcademy.com

To my family and friends, whose unwavering support fueled this journey.

To those battling type 2 diabetes, may this book guide you to lasting health.

DISCLAIMER

The content in this book is provided "as is" without any warranties, express or implied, including but not limited to merchantability, fitness for a specific purpose, or non-infringement. The authors and publishers are not liable for any loss or damage, whether direct or indirect, arising from the use of this book's information. This book offers general guidance on managing type 2 diabetes and is not a substitute for professional medical advice. Readers are strongly encouraged to consult qualified healthcare professionals before implementing any strategies or recommendations provided herein.

Table of Contents

Preface

When I was a child growing up in a bustling town in northern India, my grandfather—an energetic, cheerful man—would often rise before dawn, tie his shoes, and walk briskly through the fields. He'd return home with a smile and a handful of fresh spinach or fenugreek leaves, singing the praises of nature's bounty. But in his late sixties, his lively gait slowed, his eyes dulled, and his laughter waned. The culprit was type 2 diabetes—a diagnosis that, at the time, seemed both mysterious and inevitable.

Watching my grandfather struggle, first with fatigue and thirst, then with the side effects of medications and dietary restrictions, left a lasting imprint on my mind. Across continents and cultures, millions face the daily challenges of managing type 2 diabetes. Each diagnosis brings not only health concerns, but also social stigma, financial burdens, and emotional upheaval. Yet, amidst these challenges, I have witnessed stories of hope, resilience, and—even more remarkably—reversal.

Reverse Type 2 Diabetes Fast: A Proven Path to Lasting Health was born from a confluence of personal experience, professional inquiry, and a deep commitment to empowering others. My aim is to provide a concise, compassionate, and evidence-based roadmap for anyone seeking to take control of their health—whether you are newly diagnosed, supporting a loved one, or simply curious about the latest in diabetes management.

Motivations: Personal, Cultural, and Intellectual

My journey to writing this book is rooted in a profound respect for the intersection of tradition and science. In India, community meals, spiritual fasting, and farmers' markets are all woven into the fabric of daily life. Yet, as urbanization and westernization have changed dietary patterns worldwide, the rates of type 2 diabetes have soared—not just in India, but in America, China, the Middle East, and beyond. I have seen firsthand how cultural beliefs, family dynamics, and access to resources influence both the risk of developing diabetes and the strategies people use to manage it.

Intellectually, I have been driven by a desire to bridge the gap between cutting-edge medical research and practical, everyday wisdom. Too often, scientific findings are buried in academic journals, inaccessible to those who need them most. Conversely, misinformation abounds online and in popular media, leading to confusion and frustration. This book seeks to cut through the noise, distilling complex concepts into actionable steps while honoring the diversity of human experience.

Intended Audience

This book is written for a broad audience: from health enthusiasts eager to optimize their well-being, to individuals and families grappling with the realities of type 2 diabetes, to general readers interested in understanding one of the most pressing health challenges of our time. Whether you are a busy professional in New York, a homemaker in Cairo, a retiree in Sydney, or a student in São Paulo, my hope is that you will find both clarity and inspiration in these pages.

Unique Contribution

What sets this book apart is its unwavering commitment to accessibility, cultural sensitivity, and empowerment. While many resources focus narrowly on diet or medication, this guide embraces the complexity of diabetes reversal—addressing physical, emotional, and social dimensions. By providing tailored advice for vegetarians and incorporating global perspectives—from the Mediterranean's olive oil traditions to the rising popularity of plant-based eating in South-East Asia—this book speaks to the varied realities of readers worldwide.

I am acutely aware of the societal and historical gaps that persist in diabetes care. Language barriers, healthcare disparities, and cultural taboos can hinder progress. Here, I strive to honor those differences, offering strategies that are adaptable, inclusive, and respectful of individual journeys.

Looking Forward

As you turn these pages, remember: reversing type 2 diabetes is not a race, nor is it a solitary endeavor. It is a path—sometimes winding, often challenging, but always illuminated by the experiences of those who have walked it before. My hope is that this book will be your trusted companion, offering guidance, encouragement, and a sense of community.

May you find in these pages not only answers, but hope. The journey to reversing type 2 diabetes begins with a single, empowered step. Let us take it together.

— Rajender Kumar

Acknowledgements

Bringing **Reverse Type 2 Diabetes Fast: A Proven Path to Lasting Health** from concept to reality has been a journey marked by collaboration, insight, and unwavering support. This book would not exist without the dedication and expertise of many individuals whose contributions enriched its every page.

First, I extend my deepest gratitude to the **medical researchers and clinicians** whose groundbreaking work forms the backbone of this book. Dr. Hema Patel, your rigorous analysis of global dietary studies provided the evidence base that shaped the nutritional recommendations within these chapters. I am profoundly thankful for the **historians and archivists** who unearthed the stories and data that bring context and humanity to the science.

To my editorial team, your keen eyes and thoughtful feedback transformed complex concepts into accessible, engaging prose. Your dedication to clarity and narrative flow was instrumental in making this book both informative and inviting.

My appreciation extends to the **cultural consultants** who guided the book's inclusivity and relevance. Amit Kumar, your insights on plant-based nutrition in Middle Eastern and North African cultures helped tailor advice for diverse readers, ensuring that the book speaks to a wide audience, regardless of dietary tradition or background. Thank you for ensuring that no reader feels left behind.

Personal supporters have been the quiet strength behind this endeavor. My family—my partner and our children, your patience, understanding, and heartfelt encouragement fueled my perseverance. Friends and colleagues, especially those who shared their own stories of managing type 2 diabetes, reminded me daily of the real lives touched by this work.

Reflecting on the book's development, I am humbled by the collaborative spirit that shaped its pages. Each contributor's unique perspective—be it scientific, historical, editorial, or personal—enriched the narrative, broadened its scope, and deepened its relevance. Together, we have crafted a guide that not only informs but also empowers, offering hope and practical strategies to readers around the world.

To everyone who walked this path with me, thank you. Your commitment and generosity made this book possible and, I hope, will inspire lasting health and change for many.

Introduction

A Modern Epidemic with Ancient Roots

On a brisk autumn morning in 1946, a young physician named Dr. Elliott Joslin walked through the crowded wards of Boston's New England Deaconess Hospital. He paused at the bedside of Mary, a woman in her early forties. Mary's story mirrored that of countless others across the world: fatigue, unexplained thirst, vision problems. She had just been diagnosed with type 2 diabetes—a disease that, even then, was beginning to rise in prevalence. Dr. Joslin, a pioneer in diabetes care, believed passionately that with knowledge and discipline, his patients could reclaim their lives. "The person with diabetes who knows the most, lives the longest," he told Mary, offering hope in a time of uncertainty.

Fast forward to the 21st century, and type 2 diabetes has become a defining health crisis of our era. According to the World Health Organization, over 420 million people are living with diabetes worldwide, with type 2 diabetes accounting for the vast majority of cases. This number has nearly quadrupled since 1980—a staggering statistic that underscores the urgency of our moment. Yet, despite decades of medical advances, millions continue to struggle with the daily burdens of medication, dietary confusion, and the looming threat of complications.

But what if the story didn't have to end there? What if, armed with the right strategies, individuals could not only manage but, in many cases, reverse type 2 diabetes—restoring vitality, reducing medication, and reclaiming lasting health? This book is a guide for anyone ready to embark on that transformative journey.

Why This Book—and Why Now?

Type 2 diabetes is not merely a personal diagnosis; it is a societal phenomenon shaped by culture, history, and shifting lifestyles. From traditional diets in rural India to the fast-food revolution in North America, the ways we eat, move, and live have evolved dramatically over the past century. In the shadow of these changes, diabetes has surged—a silent epidemic that knows no borders.

Consider the case of Japan, a nation that for centuries enjoyed some of the world's lowest rates of type 2 diabetes. As post-war prosperity ushered in Western dietary habits—more processed foods, more sugar, and less physical activity—rates soared. By the early 2000s, Japan's diabetes prevalence had caught up with Western countries, starkly illustrating the profound impact of lifestyle shifts on disease.

Yet, amidst this global challenge, hope persists. Across continents and cultures, individuals and communities are discovering new ways to fight back against type 2 diabetes—through food, movement, and mindset. This book draws on these diverse stories, weaving together scientific research, real-world case studies, and actionable strategies to empower you on your path to lasting health.

The Stakes: Beyond Blood Sugar

The consequences of type 2 diabetes reach far beyond high blood sugar. It is a leading cause of heart disease, kidney failure, blindness, and limb amputations worldwide. The emotional toll is equally profound: anxiety, frustration, and the feeling of being trapped by a diagnosis. Yet, too often, conventional care focuses narrowly on medication—treating the symptoms, but rarely addressing the root causes.

Recent scientific breakthroughs have shifted the paradigm. We now know that type 2 diabetes is not an inevitable, irreversible decline. With targeted interventions—especially in the early stages—many people can put their diabetes into remission, reduce or even eliminate medications, and regain control over their health. This book is your roadmap to doing just that.

The Book's Mission and Unique Perspective

Reverse Type 2 Diabetes Fast: A Proven Path to Lasting Health is more than a manual—it is an invitation to rethink what is possible. Grounded in the latest evidence, this guide is practical, accessible, and hopeful. It recognizes that each person's journey is unique, shaped by culture, values, and life circumstances. You'll find strategies tailored for different dietary preferences—including dedicated guidance for vegetarians—and adaptable to various lifestyles.

This book is not about quick fixes or miracle cures. Instead, it champions sustainable, expert-backed habits that empower you to take charge—whether you are newly diagnosed, have lived with diabetes for years, or are seeking to prevent it altogether.

Real Stories, Real Change

The journey to reversing type 2 diabetes is as diverse as humanity itself. Consider Fatima, a grandmother in Morocco, who transformed her health by returning to the traditional couscous and vegetable stews of her youth—swapping sugary sodas for mint tea, and rediscovering the joys of walking with friends. Or Joseph, a retired teacher in the American Midwest, who found renewed energy by joining a local community garden and learning to cook with whole grains and fresh produce for the first time.

These stories remind us that change is possible, regardless of age, background, or circumstance. Across continents, people are reclaiming agency over their health—one meal, one step, one day at a time.

The Global Context: Lessons from Around the World

Type 2 diabetes is a global challenge, but solutions can be found in the lived experiences of different cultures:

The Mediterranean Paradox: Despite a diet rich in oils and carbohydrates, Mediterranean populations have historically enjoyed low rates of diabetes and heart disease. The secret? Fresh vegetables, legumes, whole grains, and physical activity woven into daily life.

The Blue Zones: In regions like Okinawa, Japan, and Nicoya, Costa Rica—where people routinely live into their nineties—traditional diets and active lifestyles have kept chronic diseases, including diabetes, at bay.

Urbanization in China: Rapid economic growth has brought dramatic dietary changes in China, with a corresponding rise in type 2 diabetes. Yet, rural communities that maintain traditional eating patterns continue to experience far lower rates of disease.

By learning from these global examples, we can craft personalized approaches that honor both scientific evidence and cultural heritage.

Your Role in the Story

Reversing type 2 diabetes is not just a medical challenge—it is a personal and societal opportunity. Whether you are living with diabetes, supporting a loved one, or seeking to prevent it in your family, your actions matter. The path ahead will require commitment, curiosity, and compassion—for yourself and for others.

This book is designed as a companion on that journey. It is structured to be practical, evidence-based, and respectful of diverse backgrounds. You will find not only the "what" and the "why," but also the "how"—tools, recipes, routines, and checklists to guide you every step of the way.

Begin Today

Mary, the patient Dr. Joslin counseled decades ago, did not have access to the knowledge, resources, or community support that we enjoy today. Yet her story, and those of countless others, remind us that with determination and the right guidance, transformation is possible.

The epidemic of type 2 diabetes need not define our future. By understanding the roots of the disease, embracing proven strategies, and honoring our own unique journeys, we can chart a new course—one of vitality, hope, and lasting health.

As you turn the page, remember: the power to reverse type 2 diabetes lies within you. Let this book be your guide, your coach, and your inspiration. The journey begins now—one choice, one meal, one step at a time.

About the Author

Rajender Kumar is a seasoned data professional whose career has spanned more than ten years at the intersection of technology, health analytics, and evidence-based decision-making. With a robust academic foundation in computer science and applied statistics, Rajender has spent his professional life translating complex data into actionable insights for global organizations, healthcare providers, and public health initiatives. His expertise extends beyond pure numbers; Rajender possesses a unique gift for drawing human stories from digital patterns, and it is this rare combination of analytical rigor and empathetic understanding that makes his work both authoritative and deeply personal.

Born in a small town in northern India, Rajender's early exposure to the cultural tapestry of health, tradition, and food shaped his worldview. In his family and community, he witnessed firsthand the silent rise of type 2 diabetes—a condition that transcended generations, economic backgrounds, and urban-rural divides. The disease was more than a medical diagnosis; it was a force that shaped daily life, family meals, and community gatherings. Rajender's own grandfather received a type 2 diabetes diagnosis in his early sixties, sparking a journey of trial, error, and eventual transformation that deeply affected the family. Navigating the maze of dietary advice, medical appointments, and cultural expectations, Rajender became the family's "data detective"—tracking blood sugar fluctuations, experimenting with food choices, and researching the latest scientific findings.

This personal odyssey ignited Rajender's passion for understanding the societal and historical dynamics of type 2 diabetes, particularly in communities where traditional diets and lifestyles were rapidly changing in the face of modernization. As he advanced in his career, Rajender recognized the urgent need for clear, culturally relevant, and evidence-based guidance to help people reclaim their health. Drawing from his professional experience analyzing global health data, he began to see patterns: the success stories from Mediterranean regions, where fresh produce and communal meals fostered resilience against diabetes; the plant-based traditions in South Asia that, when adapted thoughtfully, could offer a powerful tool for blood sugar control; and the innovative public health approaches in Scandinavia, where lifestyle medicine was transforming lives.

Rajender's unique perspective—rooted in both lived experience and analytical expertise—forms the backbone of Reverse Type 2 Diabetes Fast: A Proven Path to Lasting Health. He weaves together scientific research, cross-cultural wisdom, and practical strategies, making the book an accessible, inspiring resource for anyone seeking to understand and manage type 2 diabetes. His writing demystifies complex concepts like the glycemic index, glycemic load, and the role of plant-based nutrition, always with an eye toward sustainability and cultural sensitivity.

Above all, Rajender is driven by a belief that knowledge should empower. He is committed to breaking down barriers—whether linguistic, cultural, or scientific—to ensure that everyone has the tools to reclaim their health. Through his writing, public speaking, and community outreach, Rajender aspires to inspire lasting change, helping readers transform not only their blood sugar numbers but their entire approach to wellness. For Rajender, reversing type 2 diabetes is not just a clinical goal; it is a journey of rediscovery, resilience, and hope—a journey he is honored to share with readers worldwide.

"Let food be thy medicine and medicine be thy food—for in every bite lies the power to heal, reclaim, and transform our health."

— Rajender Kumar

A Wake-Up Call in the Waiting Room

The fluorescent lights in the clinic waiting room flickered overhead, casting a sterile glow across the sea of anxious faces. It was a Tuesday—one of those days that seem to blend into the next—when Maria, a retired schoolteacher from San Antonio, sat fidgeting with her wedding ring, her mind racing. At 62, she was no stranger to doctor's visits, but today felt different. Her blood sugar numbers had been creeping upward for years, and she'd always assumed a few pills would keep things in check. But now her doctor's words echoed in her mind: "If we don't change course, we may need to talk about insulin." She wondered how she'd gotten here—and whether it was too late to turn back.

Maria's story is not unique—it is echoed in millions of homes, clinics, and communities around the world. Type 2 diabetes, once a rare and mysterious diagnosis, has now become so common that it touches nearly every family, regardless of culture, background, or geography. Yet, for much of history, this was not the case.

The Diabetes Divide: A Tale of Two Worlds

In the early twentieth century, type 2 diabetes was known as a disease of affluence—something seen mostly in wealthier countries or among the well-to-do. In 1949, the celebrated British physician Harold Himsworth made a startling observation: in rural India, type 2 diabetes was "remarkably rare," compared to the growing epidemic in Western Europe and North America. Traditional diets—rich in legumes, whole grains, and vegetables—seemed to protect against the disease, even in the absence of modern medications or advanced healthcare.

Contrast this with the present day, where type 2 diabetes is rising faster in India and China than almost anywhere else. The shift from home-cooked meals to highly processed foods, combined with more sedentary lifestyles, has led to a dramatic increase in diabetes rates. In Mexico, the introduction of sugary sodas and convenience foods has changed the health landscape—today, more than 10% of the adult population lives with type 2 diabetes, and the nation has declared a public health emergency.

These stories—of Maria, of changing global diets, of medical breakthroughs and setbacks—are not just statistics or headlines. They are a call to action, a reminder that while our circumstances may differ, we share a common challenge. And, perhaps most importantly, we share the potential for change.

A Personal Turning Point

For many, the moment of diagnosis is a shock. For others, it comes as a slow realization—a nagging sense that something isn't right. For James, a software engineer in London, it was a routine eye exam that changed everything. "You have early signs of diabetic retinopathy," his doctor told him, explaining that high blood sugar was beginning to damage the tiny vessels in his eyes. James had always prided himself on his sharp mind, his ability to solve problems. Now, faced with a problem inside his own body, he felt powerless.

But James's story didn't end there. Driven by a desire to reclaim his health, he began researching evidence-based strategies, from dietary changes to exercise routines. He discovered that his daily choices—what he ate, how often he moved, how well he slept—could make a profound difference. Over the course of a year, with the support of his family and healthcare team, James saw his blood sugar levels normalize. His doctor marveled at his progress, and James realized he'd done something truly remarkable: he'd taken control of his health, and in doing so, had reversed the trajectory of his disease.

A New Understanding: Beyond Medication

For decades, the conventional wisdom held that type 2 diabetes was a progressive disease—manageable, perhaps, but ultimately irreversible. Medications could slow its advance, but the underlying processes seemed inexorable. Yet, as research from around the world has shown, this narrative is incomplete. In recent years, studies from the United Kingdom, the United States, Japan, and beyond have demonstrated that type 2 diabetes can, in many cases, be reversed—often through lifestyle changes alone.

In 2011, the groundbreaking DiRECT (Diabetes Remission Clinical Trial) study in the UK revealed that a structured program of dietary change and weight loss led to remission in nearly half of participants after one year. These findings echoed earlier research from Japan, where traditional diets rich in fish, soy, and vegetables were linked to lower rates of diabetes—even among those with a strong genetic predisposition.

It turns out that our bodies are more adaptable than we once believed. With the right tools, support, and information, many people can not only manage their diabetes but actually reverse its course—restoring health, vitality, and hope in the process.

A Global Challenge, A Personal Journey

Type 2 diabetes does not discriminate. It affects people of every race, religion, and economic background. In the United States, African American, Hispanic, and Native American communities face disproportionately high rates, shaped by a complicated interplay of genetics, history, access to healthcare, and social determinants. Meanwhile, in the Pacific Islands, diabetes has reached crisis levels following the loss of traditional foodways and the influx of imported processed foods. Yet, across these diverse settings, stories of resilience, adaptation, and healing abound.

The journey to reverse type 2 diabetes is not the same for everyone. Cultural traditions, family recipes, and community support all play a role. In rural Ghana, a return to millet porridge and leafy greens has helped some villages stem the tide of the disease. In urban Japan, programs that blend modern medicine with ancient food wisdom have shown promising results. In the United States, community gardens and walking groups are empowering individuals to reclaim their health, one meal and one step at a time.

Setting the Stage for Lasting Health

This book is inspired by these stories—by the urgent need for hope and clarity in a world where the problem of type 2 diabetes can feel overwhelming. It is grounded in the latest scientific research, yet it is also a practical guide, designed to empower you with tools you can use today. We will explore the intricate science of blood sugar, the powerful impact of food choices, and the ways that movement, sleep, and stress shape our bodies from the inside out. You will find tailored advice for vegetarians, strategies for embracing plant-based eating, and real-world examples from diverse cultures.

But above all, this book is a testament to possibility. Whether you are facing a new diagnosis, supporting a loved one, or simply seeking to understand this complex condition, you are not alone. The path to lasting health is not always easy, but it is within reach—one informed choice at a time.

As you turn the page, you will embark on a journey rooted in science, enriched by global perspectives, and illuminated by the stories of those who have walked this path before. Together, we will explore how to reverse type 2 diabetes—quickly, sustainably, and with a renewed sense of hope.

Laying the Foundation: Essential Resources, Mindset, and Preparatory Steps

Understanding the Journey Ahead

Before embarking on the path to reversing type 2 diabetes, it's important to recognize that this journey is as much about mindset and readiness as it is about medical facts and nutritional strategies. This book is designed to be accessible to everyone—regardless of background, age, or where you are on your health journey. Whether you've just been diagnosed, have been living with diabetes for years, or are supporting a loved one, you'll find actionable steps and encouragement within these pages.

Let's begin by outlining what you truly need—and what you don't—to make the most of the insights, advice, and inspiration this book offers.

What You Don't Need

It's natural to wonder if you need a background in medicine, a collection of specialized kitchen gadgets, or access to expensive programs to benefit from this book. The answer is a resounding no.

No prior medical or academic knowledge required: All concepts are explained in clear, everyday language. Medical terms are defined as needed, and scientific principles are broken down with relatable examples.

No specialized equipment: While some tools (like a basic glucose meter) can be helpful, you don't need a top-of-the-line kitchen, pricey supplements, or gym memberships.

No rigid rules: This book respects cultural, dietary, and lifestyle differences, offering flexible approaches that can be tailored to your individual needs.

The focus is on empowering you with knowledge and practical tools, not burdening you with unnecessary complexity.

Essential Resources: What Will Help You Thrive

1. An Open and Curious Mind

Perhaps the most important resource is a willingness to learn and try new things. Approaching your health with curiosity invites discovery and helps you move past frustration or fear.

Example: When you read about the glycemic index and glycemic load, you might initially feel overwhelmed by new terminology. Instead, view these as tools that can unlock better blood sugar control and more food enjoyment, rather than as rules to memorize. Curiosity leads you to explore how different foods affect your energy and wellbeing.

2. A Support System

Change is easier—and often more enjoyable—when shared. Support can come from family, friends, healthcare providers, or online communities.

Example: In Japan, community walking groups have helped thousands of older adults manage diabetes through collective motivation and shared accountability. You don't need a formal group; even one friend or an online forum can offer encouragement, recipe ideas, or a compassionate ear when challenges arise.

3. A Basic Toolkit for Self-Monitoring

Tracking your progress is empowering. At its simplest, this means a notebook or a free smartphone app to log meals, activity, and blood sugar readings.

Free alternatives: Many free apps, such as MyFitnessPal or Glucose Buddy, provide easy ways to monitor your food choices and glucose levels. If you prefer pen and paper, a simple diary works just as well. The goal is awareness, not perfection.

4. Time and Patience

Lasting change does not happen overnight. Set aside a few minutes daily—perhaps after breakfast or before bed—to read, reflect, and plan. Small, consistent actions compound over time.

Example: In India, community health workers support people with diabetes by encouraging "micro-changes": drinking more water, taking short walks, or swapping white rice for lentils. Each small step, repeated regularly, is a powerful investment in your long-term health.

Nurturing the Right Mindset

The way you approach this book—and your health—matters deeply. Here are three key attitudes that will enrich your experience:

Embrace Progress, Not Perfection

No one reverses type 2 diabetes in a single leap. There will be days of victory and days of challenge. Celebrate small wins and learn from setbacks.

Example: Maria, a teacher in Mexico City, started by replacing sugary drinks with infused water. She didn't change everything at once but built confidence with each small step. Her story, echoed throughout the world, reminds us that consistency matters more than intensity.

Practice Self-Compassion

Self-criticism erodes motivation. Instead, treat yourself as you would a close friend: with patience, kindness, and encouragement.

> **Example:** If you enjoy a treat at a family celebration, don't dwell on guilt. Instead, observe how it affects your body and choices, then return to your new habits. Every experience is an opportunity to learn, not a reason for shame.

Value Your Unique Context

Your culture, family traditions, and personal preferences matter. This book offers flexible strategies, recognizing that there's no one-size-fits-all solution.

> **Example:** For vegetarians in the UK and India alike, plant-based nutrition strategies are tailored to fit familiar foods and cooking methods. You'll find options that respect your values and local resources, making change feel natural and sustainable.

Accessible Alternatives: Removing Barriers

To ensure everyone can benefit, this book highlights low-cost or free options for every recommendation:

> **Exercise:** No gym required. Walking, dancing, or home-based routines are celebrated. In Cuba, for example, community squares become impromptu exercise spaces every evening.
> **Healthy eating:** Strategies focus on affordable ingredients—beans, lentils, seasonal produce—rather than expensive "superfoods."
> **Education:** All advice is grounded in accessible science, and further resources are suggested that are free or low-cost online.

Putting It All Together

In summary, the best preparation for this journey is an open mind, a willingness to explore, and a dash of patience. You don't need a medical degree or a fancy kitchen. What you do need is curiosity, a basic way to monitor your progress, and a supportive environment—whether that's a family member, an online group, or simply your own determination.

Type 2 diabetes is a global challenge, but the solutions are personal, practical, and within your reach. As you move forward through this book, remember: You are not alone, and every step you take brings you closer to lasting health.

By starting with the right resources and mindset, you pave the way for real transformation. The chapters ahead will build on this foundation—guiding you through nutrition, exercise, stress management, and more—each tailored to support your unique journey toward reversing type 2 diabetes and reclaiming vibrant health.

What You Will Gain from This Book

A Roadmap to Reclaiming Health

Embarking on the journey to reverse type 2 diabetes can feel daunting, but this book, **Reverse Type 2 Diabetes Fast: A Proven Path to Lasting Health**, is designed as your trusted companion—equipping you with the knowledge, tools, and confidence to transform your health story. Throughout these pages, you will discover not only the scientific foundations of diabetes management but also the practical wisdom and personal empowerment needed to make lasting change.

Insights and Knowledge You Will Acquire

At the heart of this book lies a clear, accessible explanation of what type 2 diabetes is, how it develops, and why it has become a global health challenge. You will learn:

The biological mechanisms that drive insulin resistance and elevated blood sugar.

Key risk factors—from genetics to lifestyle—and how they interact.

Symptoms and warning signs that often go overlooked.

Global and historical perspectives on diabetes prevalence and management.

By grounding you in a solid understanding of the condition, this book ensures that every strategy and recommendation is rooted in context—not just rules to follow, but reasons to believe.

Evidence-Based Strategies for Lasting Change

You will gain a detailed, scientifically-backed framework for managing—and, for many, potentially reversing—type 2 diabetes. This includes:

Dietary mastery, with a deep dive into the glycemic index and glycemic load, empowering you to make informed food choices.

Exercise routines tailored to different fitness levels and cultural contexts, illustrating how movement can become a joyful, sustainable part of daily life.

Stress reduction techniques and lifestyle modifications that address the emotional and psychological dimensions of diabetes.

Plant-based and vegetarian approaches, acknowledging the diversity of dietary preferences and cultural traditions.

Each of these pillars is woven together with actionable guidance, sample meal plans, and real-world stories, so you can adapt the advice to your unique circumstances.

Cultural and Historical Perspectives

Type 2 diabetes is not a one-size-fits-all problem—and its solutions are equally diverse. This book draws from a tapestry of global experiences, recognizing that cultural habits and histories shape the way we eat, move, and heal. For instance:

You will learn how **traditional Asian diets**, rich in whole grains, legumes, and vegetables, have historically kept diabetes rates low, and how these principles can be adapted for modern life.

The book examines the rise of diabetes in **Indigenous populations**—such as Native Americans and Australian Aboriginals—following shifts from ancestral diets to Westernized eating patterns, highlighting the importance of cultural food sovereignty and community-based solutions.

In a chapter dedicated to **plant-based nutrition**, you will find stories of individuals from the Mediterranean, South Asia, and Latin America who have reclaimed health by returning to time-honored, plant-forward cuisines.

A Holistic Approach to Wellness

Beyond blood sugar numbers, this book encourages you to see diabetes reversal as a pathway to holistic well-being—encompassing physical vitality, emotional resilience, and social connection. You will explore:

Mindful eating practices that foster a healthier relationship with food.

Building supportive networks—from family involvement to peer support groups—to sustain motivation.

Navigating healthcare systems and advocating for your needs, no matter where you are in the world.

Every strategy presented is sensitive to age, gender, cultural background, and individual life circumstances, ensuring inclusivity and respect for diversity.

Applying Insights in Daily Life

The knowledge you gain here is not academic theory—it is meant to be lived. Whether you are newly diagnosed, supporting a loved one, or seeking prevention, the lessons from this book can be directly applied in personal, cultural, and intellectual domains.

Community Empowerment: The Native Hawaiian Experience

In Hawaii, community-led initiatives have revived native crops like taro and breadfruit, replacing processed foods that contributed to rising diabetes rates. By reconnecting with their culinary heritage and engaging in group physical activities (like hula dancing and outrigger canoeing), participants have not only improved metabolic health but also strengthened cultural pride and social bonds. This book draws on such examples to show how collective action can amplify individual efforts.

Intellectual Curiosity: Rethinking Diabetes in the Modern World

Finally, this book challenges prevailing narratives about type 2 diabetes as an inevitable, irreversible condition. Through a blend of history, science, and real-life success stories, it invites readers to reconsider what is possible. You will be encouraged to ask new questions, explore diverse perspectives, and become an informed advocate for yourself and your community.

Relevance to Today's Societal Conversations

The prevalence of type 2 diabetes has reached historic heights, touching millions of lives worldwide and straining healthcare systems. In many regions, the condition is intertwined with issues of food access, socioeconomic inequality, and cultural identity. This book is timely—addressing urgent questions:

- How do we respect traditional foodways while embracing modern science?
- What does it mean to reverse diabetes in a world of rapid urbanization and global food marketing?
- How can individuals reclaim agency over their health amidst often conflicting messages from media and medicine?

By engaging with these themes, you are joining a larger, global conversation about health, justice, and the future of our communities.

Rajender Kumar

REVERSE TYPE 2 DIABETES FAST

A Proven Path to Lasting Health

1 : Understanding Type 2 Diabetes – The Global Epidemic

1.1 The Rise of Type 2 Diabetes Worldwide

When we look back just a century, **type 2 diabetes** was a rarity, often referred to as "*adult-onset diabetes*" and largely confined to wealthier nations. Now, it is a global health crisis, affecting hundreds of millions across every continent. The story of its rise is one of shifting lifestyles, traditions, and diets—a story that mirrors the dramatic changes of the modern era.

The Global Surge: A Modern Epidemic

Over the last five decades, the number of people diagnosed with type 2 diabetes has skyrocketed. According to the World Health Organization (WHO), in 1980, an estimated **108 million** adults lived with diabetes worldwide. Today, that number has soared past **500 million—over four times as many**. This rapid escalation is not limited to high-income countries; low- and middle-income nations now carry the greatest burden.

Several factors have contributed to this explosive growth:

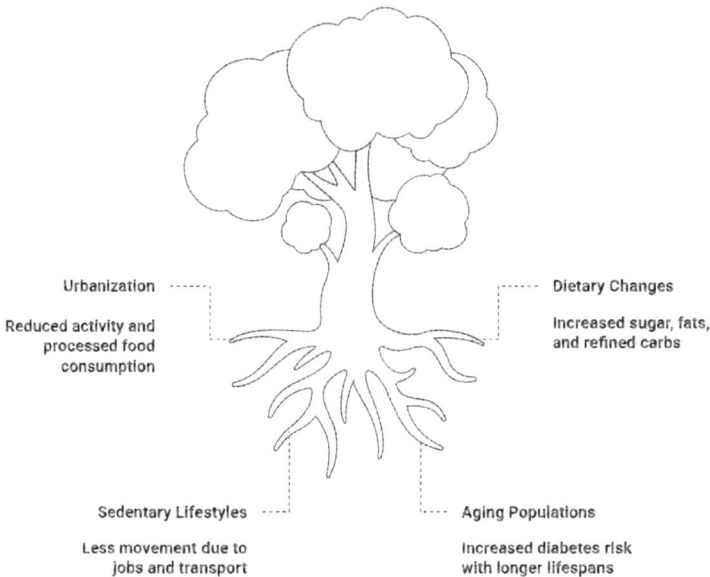

Rising Type-2 Diabetes Cases

Urbanization
Reduced activity and processed food consumption

Dietary Changes
Increased sugar, fats, and refined carbs

Sedentary Lifestyles
Less movement due to jobs and transport

Aging Populations
Increased diabetes risk with longer lifespans

- **Urbanization:** As people move from rural to urban areas, physical activity often decreases, and diets shift toward processed foods.
- **Dietary Changes:** Traditional diets rich in whole grains, legumes, and vegetables are being replaced by foods high in sugars, unhealthy fats, and refined carbohydrates.
- **Sedentary Lifestyles:** The rise of desk jobs, screen time, and mechanized transport reduces daily movement.
- **Aging Populations:** With longer life expectancies, more people are at risk of developing diabetes as they age.

The impact is staggering: type 2 diabetes is now a leading cause of heart disease, kidney failure, blindness, and lower-limb amputation globally.

Diabetes Causes Global Health Issues

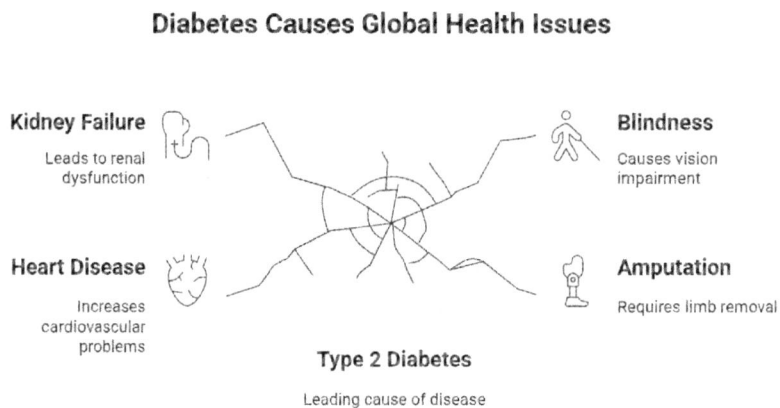

Kidney Failure
Leads to renal dysfunction

Blindness
Causes vision impairment

Heart Disease
Increases cardiovascular problems

Amputation
Requires limb removal

Type 2 Diabetes
Leading cause of disease

A Tale of Two Cities: Real-World Transformations

To understand the scope of the problem, consider the experience of two vastly different societies—one in the West, the other in the East.

In the United States, type 2 diabetes has become almost synonymous with modern lifestyle diseases. The story of **John**, a middle-aged office worker from Chicago, is emblematic. John grew up in the 1970s, when family meals were home-cooked and outdoor play was the norm. As an adult, his daily routine changed: breakfast at a drive-thru, hours seated at a computer, and little time for exercise. In his late forties, John was diagnosed with type 2 diabetes. His story is not unique—more than **1 in 10 Americans** now have diabetes, the vast majority of whom have type 2.

Contrast this with the experience of **urban India**. For much of the 20th century, diabetes was rare among Indians, whose diets centered on whole grains, lentils, and vegetables. But as cities like Mumbai and New Delhi have grown, so too has the prevalence of type 2 diabetes. **Meera**, a young professional in Mumbai, recalls her grandmother walking several miles a day and cooking fresh meals from scratch. Meera's own schedule is a whirlwind of work meetings, convenience foods, and commutes by car. She was stunned to learn, at age 32, that she was prediabetic. In India, diabetes rates have doubled in the last two decades, affecting younger and younger people.

These stories, while personal, reflect broader societal shifts. Countries undergoing rapid economic development often experience the most dramatic increases—sometimes described as a "diabetes tsunami."

Historical Context: From Scarcity to Surplus

The rise of type 2 diabetes is closely tied to historical changes in the way we live and eat. For most of human history, food was scarce, and physical labor was a daily necessity. Sugary treats and processed snacks were luxuries, not staples. Our bodies evolved to store energy efficiently, a survival advantage in lean times.

The post-World War II era marked a turning point. Advances in food processing, preservation, and transportation made calorie-dense, affordable foods widely available. Supermarkets replaced local markets; fast food chains spread globally. In many cultures, traditional meals gave way to convenience, and physical work was supplanted by machines.

A notable example is the **Pima people** of Arizona. Historically, the Pima thrived on a diet of beans, corn, and squash, combined with regular physical activity. But with the introduction of Western foods and lifestyles, diabetes rates soared—today, the Pima have one of the highest rates of type 2 diabetes in the world. Their story is a warning and a lesson: rapid lifestyle changes can dramatically affect health in just a generation.

Lifestyle Changes and Diabetes Risk

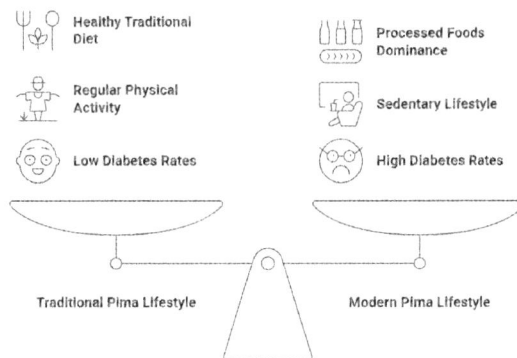

Healthy Traditional Diet		Processed Foods Dominance
Regular Physical Activity		Sedentary Lifestyle
Low Diabetes Rates		High Diabetes Rates

Traditional Pima Lifestyle · Modern Pima Lifestyle

The Numbers Behind the Crisis

Let's trace the timeline of diabetes' rise:

- **Pre-1950s:** Type 2 diabetes is rare, mostly seen in affluent, urban populations.
- **1950s–1970s:** Economic growth and urbanization begin to change diets and activity patterns, especially in Western countries.
- **1980s–2000s:** Diabetes becomes more common globally, with sharp increases in Asia, the Middle East, and Latin America.
- **2010s–Today:** Type 2 diabetes is a leading public health challenge, affecting people of all ages, ethnicities, and backgrounds.

Progression of Type 2 Diabetes

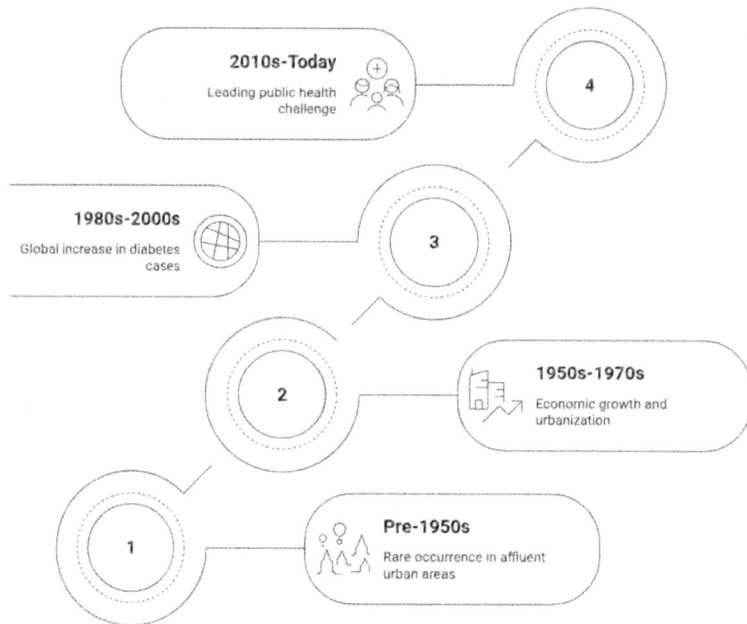

Very important fact: Over 90% of diabetes cases worldwide are type 2 diabetes, and many cases are preventable or reversible through lifestyle changes.

The rise of type 2 diabetes is not simply a medical issue—it is a reflection of how our societies, diets, and daily routines have changed. The good news is that understanding its roots allows us to take decisive action. In the next section, we will unravel what happens in the body during type 2 diabetes and how the condition develops. By grasping the science behind the epidemic, you will be better equipped to reverse its course—and reclaim your health.

1.2 What Is Type 2 Diabetes?

At the heart of **type 2 diabetes** lies a delicate dance between glucose—your body's primary energy source—and insulin, the hormone responsible for ushering that glucose from your bloodstream into your cells. In a healthy body, this process runs smoothly: after you eat, blood sugar rises, the pancreas releases insulin, and cells happily absorb the fuel they need. But in type 2 diabetes, this harmony is disrupted.

Glucose-Insulin Cycle in Type 2 Diabetes

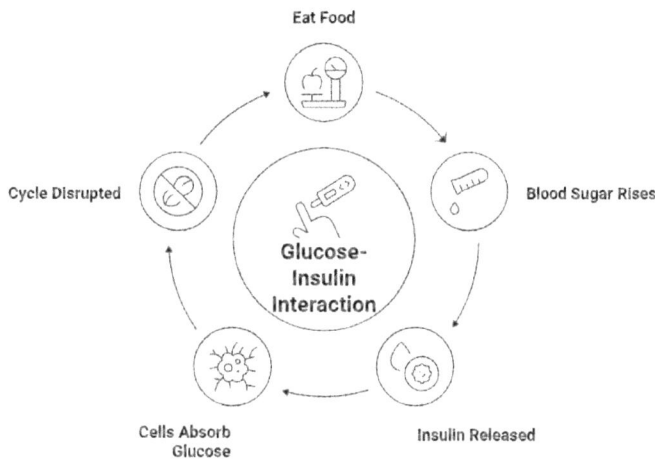

Eat Food

Blood Sugar Rises

Glucose-Insulin Interaction

Cycle Disrupted

Insulin Released

Cells Absorb Glucose

The trouble typically begins with **insulin resistance**. Your cells start to ignore insulin's signals, causing glucose to build up in your blood. The pancreas tries to compensate by pumping out even more insulin, but over time, this relentless demand exhausts the insulin-producing beta cells. Eventually, the pancreas can't keep up, and blood sugar levels climb steadily higher.

How Type 2 Diabetes Develops

Type 2 diabetes doesn't appear overnight. It's often the result of years—sometimes decades—of subtle metabolic shifts. These changes can be influenced by a variety of factors, including:

- **Genetics**: A family history of diabetes can increase your risk, but genes are only part of the story.
- **Lifestyle**: Diets high in processed foods, sedentary habits, chronic stress, and poor sleep all contribute.

- **Age**: Risk rises as we grow older, though more young people are now being diagnosed worldwide.

This gradual progression means there's a critical window for intervention. Many people first develop **prediabetes**, a condition where blood sugar is higher than normal, but not yet in the diabetic range. With targeted lifestyle changes, prediabetes—and even early-stage type 2 diabetes—can often be reversed.

The Global Impact: A Modern Epidemic

To understand the urgency of reversing type 2 diabetes, consider its staggering reach. According to the International Diabetes Federation, over **500 million people** globally live with diabetes, and the vast majority have type 2. Once considered a "disease of affluence," it now affects people in every corner of the world, from bustling cities in India to small towns in the American Midwest.

Real-World Example: India's Diabetes Paradox

India offers a striking example of this global shift. Traditional Indian diets, rich in whole grains, pulses, and vegetables, kept diabetes rates low for centuries. But as Western-style fast foods and sedentary desk jobs have proliferated, so too has type 2 diabetes. Today, India has one of the highest numbers of diabetes cases worldwide—a powerful reminder that lifestyle changes can either fuel or fight the epidemic.

Personal Story: Reclaiming Health in the Heartland

Mary's Journey to Diabetes Remission

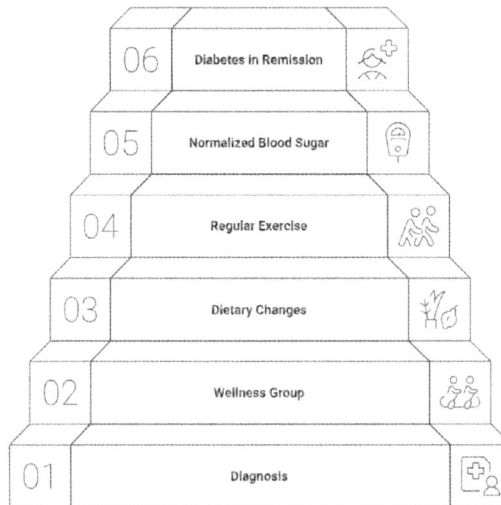

06	Diabetes in Remission
05	Normalized Blood Sugar
04	Regular Exercise
03	Dietary Changes
02	Wellness Group
01	Diagnosis

Consider the story of Mary, a grandmother from Ohio. After years of enjoying nightly desserts and minimal exercise, Mary was diagnosed with type 2 diabetes in her late fifties. Rather than resign herself to daily medications, she joined a local wellness group, swapped processed snacks for fresh produce, and began walking with friends every morning. Within a year, Mary's blood sugar normalized, and her doctor declared her diabetes "in remission." Her journey illustrates a profound truth: with the right tools, lasting change is possible.

Left unchecked, high blood sugar can damage blood vessels and nerves throughout the body, increasing the risk of heart disease, kidney failure, vision loss, and even limb amputations. Recognizing symptoms early—and acting swiftly—can mean the difference between long-term complications and a vibrant, healthy life.

The Science of Reversal: Why Hope Matters

While the statistics can seem overwhelming, research reveals a hopeful reality: **type 2 diabetes is not inevitable or irreversible**. Studies from the United Kingdom, Japan, and elsewhere have shown that targeted nutrition, regular exercise, and weight loss can restore insulin sensitivity and even induce remission in many patients. This means that, for countless people, a diagnosis is not a life sentence—it's a wake-up call and an opportunity for transformation.

```
Memorable Fact: Type 2 diabetes can often be reversed or placed into remission
through lifestyle changes, especially when addressed early.
Vital Insight: Many people live with type 2 diabetes for years before
diagnosis—early detection and intervention are crucial for reversal.
```

Type 2 diabetes is a complex but manageable condition, rooted in the interplay between genetics, lifestyle, and environment. Its global rise underscores the importance of understanding not just what diabetes is, but how it unfolds—and, crucially, how it can be reversed. In the next section, we'll explore the risk factors that lead to type 2 diabetes, empowering you to identify and address them before they become roadblocks on your path to lasting health.

1.3 Recognizing the Symptoms

For many, the journey toward reversing type 2 diabetes begins with the simple act of recognition. Understanding when your body is trying to alert you can mean the difference between early intervention and years of silent damage. The symptoms of type 2 diabetes are often subtle at first—so subtle, in fact, that millions live with undiagnosed diabetes for years. This hidden progression is part of what has fueled the global epidemic, making awareness and vigilance crucial tools in the fight for lasting health.

The Body's Early Warnings

While everyone's experience with **type 2 diabetes** is unique, a cluster of classic symptoms tends to appear as blood sugar levels rise over time. Think of these as your body's "check engine" light—a signal that something deeper may be wrong.

Type 2 Diabetes: Silent Progression

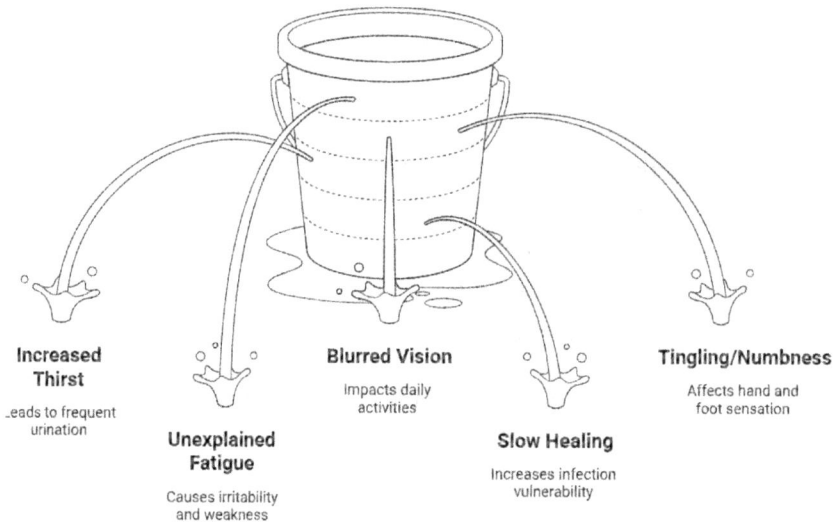

Increased Thirst
_eads to frequent urination

Unexplained Fatigue
Causes irritability and weakness

Blurred Vision
Impacts daily activities

Slow Healing
Increases infection vulnerability

Tingling/Numbness
Affects hand and foot sensation

- **Increased thirst and frequent urination:** High blood sugar draws water out of the tissues, leaving you thirsty and sending your kidneys into overdrive.
- **Fatigue:** When cells can't efficiently absorb glucose, energy levels plummet, resulting in persistent tiredness.
- **Blurred vision:** High blood sugar can cause the lenses of your eyes to swell, distorting your vision.
- **Slow-healing wounds or frequent infections:** Excess glucose impairs the immune system, making it harder for your body to recover.
- **Unexplained weight loss:** Even with normal or increased eating, your body may start breaking down muscle and fat for energy.
- **Tingling or numbness in hands or feet:** Persistently high blood sugar can damage nerves, leading to a condition called neuropathy.

A Personal Story: Maria's Wake-Up Call

Consider the story of **Maria Gutierrez**, a 48-year-old teacher from Buenos Aires. Maria had always attributed her midday fatigue to her busy classroom and her blurry vision to aging. It wasn't until a persistent foot sore refused to heal that she visited her doctor, who promptly diagnosed her with type 2 diabetes. The diagnosis was shocking, but in hindsight, Maria realized her body had been sending her subtle messages for months.

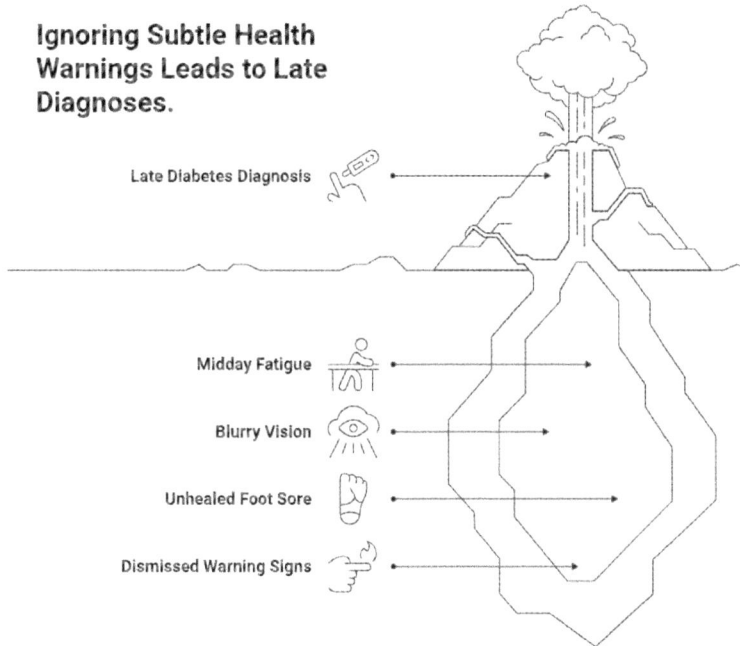

Ignoring Subtle Health Warnings Leads to Late Diagnoses.

Late Diabetes Diagnosis

Midday Fatigue

Blurry Vision

Unhealed Foot Sore

Dismissed Warning Signs

Maria's experience is not unique. All over the world, countless individuals dismiss these warning signs as the inevitable side effects of a busy life, stress, or getting older. Yet, it is exactly these small, persistent changes that demand our attention.

Timeline of Symptoms: From Subtle to Severe

Type 2 diabetes does not emerge overnight. The progression from elevated blood sugar to full-blown diabetes can take years, often following this sequence:

- **Prediabetes:** Slight increases in blood sugar with little to no symptoms.
- **Early symptoms:** Mild increases in thirst, urination, or fatigue.
- **Escalating symptoms:** Noticeable slow healing, frequent infections, vision changes.
- **Advanced symptoms:** Significant weight loss, nerve pain, or numbness.

Recognizing where you or a loved one might fall on this spectrum can be the first step toward timely intervention.

Cultural Perspectives: Recognizing Symptoms Worldwide

Awareness of diabetes symptoms varies greatly across cultures and communities. In rural India, for instance, **Asha workers** (community health volunteers) have played a pivotal role in educating villagers about the early signs of diabetes, often catching cases before complications arise. Meanwhile, in Scandinavian countries, national health campaigns have helped raise public awareness, leading to earlier detection and better outcomes.

These global examples highlight a universal truth: education and vigilance can break the pattern of silent suffering. Regardless of where you live, knowing the signs and acting on them empowers you to take control before complications develop.

Why Early Recognition Matters

Catching diabetes early doesn't just mean fewer symptoms—it can literally change your trajectory. Studies have shown that early detection and intervention can prevent or delay the need for lifelong medication, reduce the risk of complications, and, in many cases, set the stage for successful reversal.

Very Important: Up to 1 in 2 people with type 2 diabetes are unaware they have it—early recognition is essential for reversal.

Taking Action: What to Do If You Suspect Diabetes

If you recognize any of these symptoms in yourself or a loved one, consider these steps:

- Schedule a check-up with your healthcare provider for a blood sugar test.
- Keep a symptom diary to track any changes over time.
- Discuss your family history and lifestyle factors with your doctor.

Early intervention not only improves prognosis but can also make the path to reversal less daunting.

Recognizing the symptoms of type 2 diabetes is a powerful act of self-care—one that bridges the gap between silent suffering and proactive health. By listening to our bodies and understanding the signals they send, we set ourselves up for success on the journey to reversal. In the coming section, we'll delve into the risk factors that pave the way for type 2 diabetes, equipping you with knowledge to prevent or halt its progression before symptoms even arise.

1.4 The Science of Blood Sugar

At the heart of type 2 diabetes lies a deceptively simple molecule: **glucose**, commonly referred to as blood sugar. Glucose is the body's primary energy currency, fueling everything from brain function to muscle contractions. After eating, our digestive system breaks down carbohydrates into glucose, which then enters the bloodstream. This surge in blood sugar signals the pancreas to release **insulin**—a hormone that acts as a gatekeeper, allowing cells to absorb and use glucose for energy.

But what happens when this finely tuned system falters? In type 2 diabetes, the body's cells become resistant to insulin's effects, or the pancreas can't produce enough insulin to keep up. Blood sugar remains elevated, silently damaging blood vessels, nerves, and organs over time.

The Insulin-Glucose Dance

To fully grasp how type 2 diabetes develops, it's helpful to visualize the **insulin-glucose dance**:

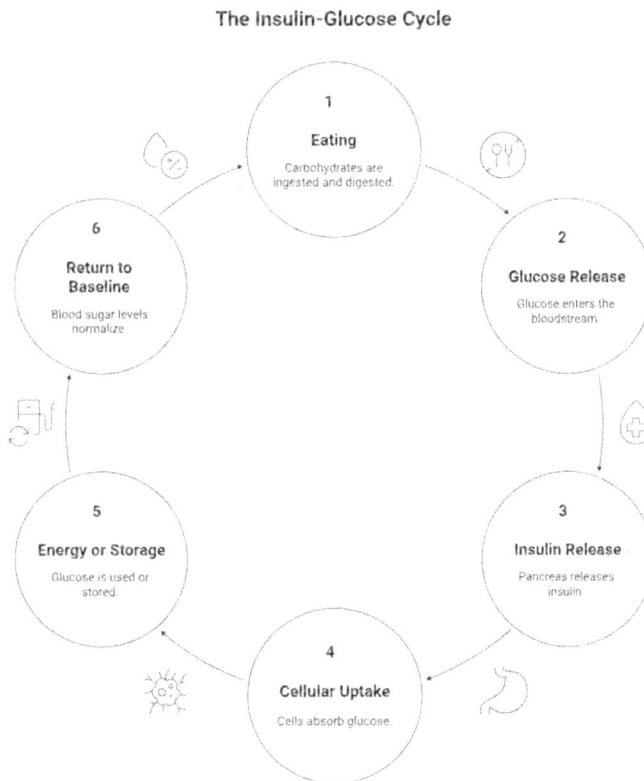

The Insulin-Glucose Cycle

- **Eating:** Carbohydrates are ingested and digested, releasing glucose into the blood.

- **Insulin Release:** The pancreas detects rising glucose and releases insulin.
- **Cellular Uptake:** Insulin "unlocks" cells so they can absorb glucose.
- **Energy or Storage:** Cells use glucose for energy, or store it as glycogen in muscles and the liver.
- **Return to Baseline:** Blood sugar levels fall, and insulin release tapers.

In healthy individuals, this process keeps blood sugar within a narrow, safe range. But in type 2 diabetes, the dance becomes uncoordinated. Insulin's signal weakens, and glucose lingers in the bloodstream—a condition known as **hyperglycemia.**

How Insulin Resistance Develops

Insulin resistance doesn't happen overnight. It's often the result of years of subtle changes:

- **Excess weight, especially around the abdomen**
- **Physical inactivity**
- **Genetic predisposition**
- **Chronic stress and poor sleep**
- **Unhealthy diet high in processed foods and sugars**

As resistance escalates, the pancreas works harder, pumping out more insulin. Eventually, it can't keep up—leading to persistently high blood sugar.

The Global Impact: From Ancient Descriptions to Modern Epidemic

The story of diabetes spans centuries. Ancient Egyptian texts described excessive thirst and urination, hallmarks of what we now recognize as diabetes. In 19th-century India, physicians noticed ants being drawn to the sweet urine of people with the disease, giving rise to the term "madhumeha" (honey urine).

Fast forward to the 21st century, and type 2 diabetes has reached epidemic proportions. Once considered a disease of affluence, it now affects people in all corners of the globe—from bustling cities in the United States to rural villages in sub-Saharan Africa. For example, in Japan, the rapid adoption of Western eating habits after World War II led to a dramatic uptick in type 2 diabetes rates, demonstrating the profound impact of lifestyle on blood sugar regulation.

Conversely, even modest improvements in blood sugar can yield dramatic health benefits. Studies show that every 1% reduction in HbA1c—a marker of average blood sugar—can lower the risk of diabetes complications by up to 40%.

Insulin resistance can develop years before symptoms appear, making early lifestyle changes crucial.

- The body's normal fasting blood sugar range is typically 70-99 mg/dL (3.9-5.5 mmol/L).

1.5 The Long-Term Consequences

Type 2 diabetes is often described as a "silent" condition—not merely because its early symptoms can be subtle, but because its most profound impact unfolds slowly, over years or even decades. While the immediate challenges of high blood sugar may seem manageable at first, the true burden of diabetes lies in its long-term consequences. These outcomes touch nearly every organ system in the body, reshaping lives, families, and even entire communities.

How Type 2 Diabetes Affects the Body Over Time

Persistent high blood sugar gradually damages blood vessels and nerves, setting off a cascade of complications. Each year spent with poorly controlled diabetes increases the risk of developing serious health issues, many of which become irreversible if not addressed early.

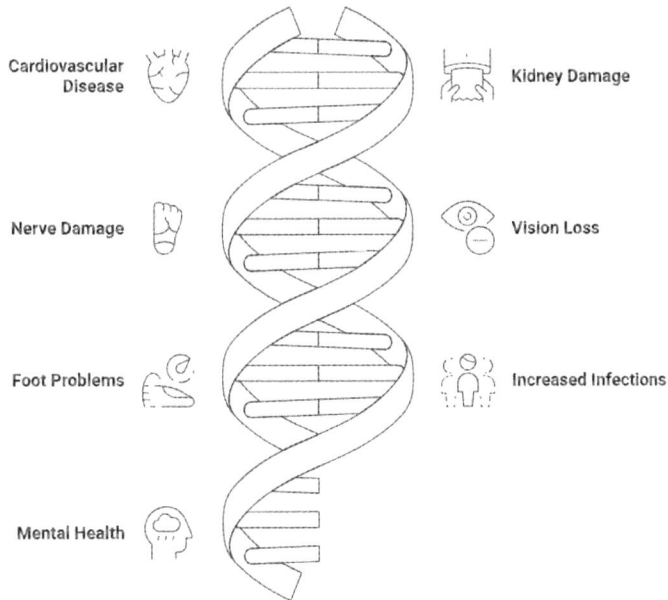

Complications of Uncontrolled Diabetes

- **Cardiovascular Disease:** Diabetes more than doubles the risk of heart attacks and strokes, as excess glucose damages arteries and accelerates the buildup of fatty plaques.

- **Kidney Damage (Nephropathy):** Over time, the kidneys' delicate filtering system becomes scarred, leading to chronic kidney disease and sometimes end-stage renal failure requiring dialysis or transplant.
- **Nerve Damage (Neuropathy):** Tingling, numbness, and pain—especially in the legs and feet—are common as nerves deteriorate. This can progress to loss of sensation, increasing the risk of unnoticed injuries.
- **Vision Loss (Retinopathy):** The tiny vessels at the back of the eye are vulnerable to high blood sugar. Diabetic retinopathy is a leading cause of blindness in adults worldwide.
- **Foot Problems:** Poor circulation and nerve damage combine to make infections and ulcers more likely. In severe cases, this can lead to amputation.
- **Increased Risk of Infections:** The immune system becomes less effective, making even minor infections potentially dangerous.
- **Mental Health:** The emotional toll of chronic illness, combined with the direct effects of blood sugar on the brain, increases the risk of depression and cognitive decline.

A Timeline of Complications

Understanding how these complications develop underscores the urgency of early and sustained intervention.

First 5 Years: Subtle nerve and blood vessel changes begin, often unnoticed. Some vision changes or mild neuropathy may appear.

5–10 Years: Risk of heart attack and stroke rises. Early kidney and eye damage may be detected on routine screening.

10+ Years: Advanced complications—such as kidney failure, significant vision loss, or major cardiovascular events—become more common, especially if blood sugar has not been well controlled.

Australia's Indigenous Communities:

In Australia, type 2 diabetes has had a devastating impact on some Indigenous communities. Rates of kidney failure are among the highest in the world, and the need for dialysis has placed enormous strain on families and healthcare systems. Community leaders and health workers are now championing culturally tailored prevention and reversal programs, emphasizing the importance of diet, exercise, and early screening to break this cycle.

The Global Toll

Globally, the number of people experiencing diabetes-related complications is staggering. According to the World Health Organization, diabetes is a leading cause of blindness, kidney failure, heart attacks, stroke, and lower limb amputation. The economic burden is equally profound, with billions spent on treating complications that, in many cases, could have been prevented.

Breaking the Cycle

The most important message for anyone living with type 2 diabetes—or at risk of developing it—is this: These outcomes are not inevitable. With timely, sustained intervention, many of the long-term consequences can be delayed, minimized, or even prevented altogether. Dietary changes, regular exercise, stress management, and medical support form the foundation of a new path—one that leads toward better health and renewed hope.

Fast Facts to Remember

- Early and aggressive management of type 2 diabetes can reduce the risk of heart disease by more than 50%.
- Vision loss from diabetic retinopathy is often preventable with regular screening and good blood sugar control.

In reflecting on the long-term consequences of type 2 diabetes, it is clear that the stakes are high, but so too is the potential for meaningful change. By understanding what's at risk, we become empowered to take action—not only for ourselves, but for our families and communities. In the next section, we'll examine the risk factors that set the stage for this condition, illuminating the choices and circumstances that can tip the balance toward either vulnerability or resilience.

1.6 Why This Book Matters

Imagine standing at a crossroads. One path leads to a future marked by uncertainty—frequent doctor visits, increasing medications, and the looming shadow of complications. The other offers the promise of renewed energy, independence, and lasting health. For millions around the globe diagnosed with type 2 diabetes, this is not a distant metaphor but a daily reality. The question is: Which path will you choose?

The Urgency Behind the Epidemic

Type 2 diabetes has evolved from a rare diagnosis to a global epidemic within a single generation. In the 1980s, only a handful of nations faced significant rates of the disease. Fast forward to today, and countries from India to the United States, from South Africa to Brazil, are grappling with surging numbers. The World Health Organization estimates that over 420 million adults are living with diabetes worldwide, the vast majority with type 2. This staggering figure is not just a testament to changing lifestyles; it's a call to action.

The consequences are profound. Unchecked, type 2 diabetes can lead to heart disease, kidney failure, vision loss, and nerve damage. The emotional toll—stress, fear, and even stigma—can be just as debilitating. Yet, amidst these challenges, an empowering truth emerges: much of the trajectory of type 2 diabetes can be shaped by informed choices.

Why a New Approach is Needed

Conventional wisdom often frames type 2 diabetes as a lifelong, progressively worsening condition. Many are told that medication is their only option, and that managing the disease means simply slowing its inevitable march. But recent scientific advances, clinical trials, and thousands of individual success stories have begun to rewrite this narrative.

- **Lifestyle interventions**—including diet, exercise, and stress management—can dramatically improve blood sugar control, sometimes even leading to remission.
- **Personalized nutrition** and the understanding of glycemic index and glycemic load have revealed that what and how we eat matters profoundly.
- **Cultural and social factors** play a significant role, underscoring the importance of tailored strategies instead of one-size-fits-all solutions.

Consider the story of Ana, a grandmother from São Paulo. Diagnosed in her early fifties, she felt overwhelmed and resigned to a lifetime of pills. But after joining a community-based nutrition and exercise program, she not only lost weight and improved her blood sugar but reduced her reliance on medications. Her journey is echoed in villages in India, where local adaptations of traditional diets and daily walks have helped entire communities turn the tide against diabetes.

What Makes This Book Different

This book stands apart because it blends the rigor of scientific research with the compassion of real-world understanding. Here's what you can expect:

- **Evidence-based guidance**: Every recommendation is rooted in the latest clinical research, not fads or quick fixes.
- **Practical strategies**: From shopping lists to sample meal plans, from beginner workouts to advanced routines, you'll find tools that fit real lives.

- **Inclusivity**: Whether you're a lifelong vegetarian, a busy parent, or someone juggling multiple health concerns, the advice here respects your culture, preferences, and needs.
- **Sustainability**: The focus is on lasting change, not temporary deprivation. You'll learn how to build habits that endure.

The Power of Choice and Community

The story of reversing or managing type 2 diabetes is not just about individual willpower. It's about harnessing the strength of community and the wisdom of collective experience. In Japan, for example, workplace wellness programs that encourage group exercise and healthy lunches have helped lower diabetes rates among employees. In the United States, support groups—both in-person and online—have become lifelines for people seeking accountability and inspiration.

As you read, you'll meet people from diverse backgrounds who reclaimed their health—not through heroic acts, but through daily, doable steps. Their successes are proof that change is possible, regardless of age, background, or past setbacks.

The Stakes and the Hope

Let's be clear: reversing type 2 diabetes fast is not about miracle cures or overnight transformations. It's about understanding your body, making informed choices, and building a life where health, not disease, takes center stage.

Type 2 diabetes is not an inevitable fate; with the right strategies, many people can achieve lasting remission and reduce or eliminate their need for medication.

The glycemic index and glycemic load are powerful tools that help you make food choices that stabilize blood sugar—key to reversing type 2 diabetes.

In the next section, we'll explore the risk factors that set the stage for type 2 diabetes, illuminating the choices and circumstances that can tip the balance toward either vulnerability or resilience. By understanding what puts us at risk, we empower ourselves to make mindful changes—setting the foundation for everything that follows.

2 : The Roots of the Problem – Causes and Risk Factors

2.1 Genetics and Family History

The story of type 2 diabetes does not begin or end with lifestyle alone. For many, the roots of this condition are entwined with family history and the invisible hand of genetics. Understanding how our DNA shapes our risk is a crucial step in the journey toward reversing and managing diabetes.

The Genetic Blueprint: Inheritance and Predisposition

The question often arises: "If my parents or grandparents had type 2 diabetes, am I destined for the same fate?" The answer is nuanced. Genetics do not seal your destiny, but they do influence the playing field.

Family history is one of the strongest risk factors for type 2 diabetes. If you have a first-degree relative (parent, sibling) with the condition, your risk can be up to three times higher than someone without that family background. Scientists have identified more than 400 genetic variants associated with type 2 diabetes, each playing a modest role in how your body processes insulin and glucose.

The Dual Path to Diabetes Development

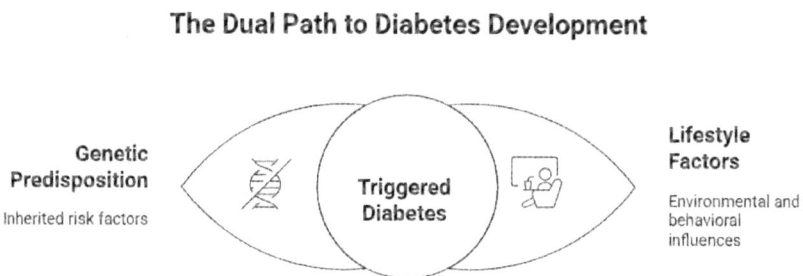

Genetic Predisposition — Inherited risk factors

Triggered Diabetes

Lifestyle Factors — Environmental and behavioral influences

However, **genetics load the gun—lifestyle pulls the trigger**. The majority of people who inherit these risk genes only develop diabetes when environmental and lifestyle factors—such as poor diet, inactivity, and chronic stress—come into play.

A Tale of Two Families: Real-World Stories

Consider the story of the Hernandez family in Texas. For generations, they struggled with weight and blood sugar issues. When Maria, the youngest daughter, was diagnosed with prediabetes at 28, she feared her path was set. Yet, Maria embarked on a journey of nutrition education, regular exercise, and stress management. Within a year, her blood sugar levels normalized, and she inspired her siblings and cousins to follow suit. Maria's story is a testament to the power of knowledge and action over genetic predisposition.

Across the globe in Mumbai, the Shah family faced a similar legacy. Rakesh, a 52-year-old accountant, watched his father and uncles succumb to diabetes-related complications. When Rakesh's blood tests revealed rising glucose levels, he chose a different path—joining a community walking group and embracing traditional, high-fiber, plant-based meals. Over time, his health markers improved, demonstrating that genes are only part of the equation.

Unpacking the Science

To understand why some families seem more susceptible, it helps to look beneath the surface:

> **Insulin resistance**—the hallmark of type 2 diabetes—can be influenced by genes that affect how fat is stored, how cells respond to insulin, and how the liver manages glucose production.
>
> Certain populations, such as South Asians, Pacific Islanders, and African Americans, have a higher genetic predisposition to insulin resistance. This has historical roots: in times of scarcity, genes that favored efficient energy storage were advantageous. In today's world of calorie abundance, these genes can backfire.

```
Remember: Having a family history of type 2 diabetes does NOT mean you cannot
prevent or reverse the condition. Lifestyle changes have a powerful impact,
even in those with high genetic risk.
```

The Rise of Genetic Testing

Advancements in genetic testing have made it possible to estimate an individual's risk for type 2 diabetes. While these tests can offer insight, they are not crystal balls. Most experts agree that knowing your family history—who in your family had diabetes and at what age—remains one of the most useful predictors.

> **Gene-environment interaction** is at the heart of diabetes risk. For example, a child with high-risk genes raised in an active, healthy-eating household may never develop diabetes. In contrast, someone with moderate risk genes but poor lifestyle habits may develop the condition much earlier.

The Intergenerational Cycle

The impact of diabetes risk can echo across generations, not only through DNA but also through family habits and culture:

Children often inherit not just genes but also eating patterns, attitudes toward exercise, and approaches to stress.

Breaking the cycle requires a conscious effort to create new family traditions—like cooking healthy meals together or taking evening walks.

Key Takeaways for Action

Know your family history and share it with your healthcare provider.

Focus on what you can control: daily choices in food, activity, and stress management.

Engage your relatives in healthful changes—success is often contagious within families.

`You are not your genes. The most powerful predictor of your future health is what you do today.`

Understanding the role of genetics and family history in type 2 diabetes is empowering, not limiting. By recognizing risk and taking proactive steps, individuals and families can rewrite their health story. In the next section, we'll explore the impact of lifestyle and environmental factors—where your choices can make all the difference.

2.2 The Modern Lifestyle

From the moment we wake to the time we sleep, modern life offers unprecedented convenience—yet beneath this ease lies a web of choices that often work against our health. The contemporary lifestyle, shaped by technology, urbanization, and shifting cultural norms, is a major driving force behind the global surge in type 2 diabetes. Understanding how these factors quietly erode our metabolic health is key to taking back control.

Sedentary Living: The Hidden Cost of Comfort

The digital revolution, while transformative in countless positive ways, has also unintentionally contributed to widespread inactivity. Work that once required physical labor now frequently happens at desks or on screens. Commuting by car, shopping online, and entertainment delivered to our couches mean many of us spend hours each day barely moving.

A striking example comes from a study in the United States, where the average adult sits for more than 10 hours a day. The result? Muscles become less efficient at using glucose, and insulin sensitivity plummets. This effect is not confined to wealthy nations; urbanization in countries like India and Brazil has led to similar patterns, with rural populations adopting city habits and seeing a corresponding rise in diabetes rates.

Processed Foods: Convenience with Consequences

Convenience foods line our supermarket shelves, offering quick solutions to our busy schedules. But these highly processed products—often rich in refined carbohydrates, added sugars, and unhealthy fats—are a major contributor to the diabetes epidemic.

Take the story of **Miguel**, a factory worker in Mexico City. Like many, Miguel found himself relying on soft drinks, packaged snacks, and fast food to fuel his long workdays. Within a decade, he joined millions of Mexicans diagnosed with type 2 diabetes, a condition now so prevalent it has been declared a national health emergency. Miguel's experience reflects a global pattern: as traditional diets rich in whole grains, legumes, and vegetables are replaced by Westernized, processed fare, rates of metabolic disease skyrocket.

The Stress Factor: When the Mind Impacts the Body

Stress is another hallmark of modern living. Whether from workplace pressures, financial worries, or the relentless pace of digital connectivity, chronic stress floods the body with hormones like cortisol. Over time, elevated cortisol levels drive up blood sugar and promote fat storage—particularly around the abdomen, a key risk factor for insulin resistance.

Consider **Yuko**, a Tokyo-based office worker, who found herself trapped in a cycle of long hours and little rest. Despite a normal body weight, her stress-induced insomnia and erratic eating patterns led to rising blood sugar levels. Her case illustrates how diabetes risk is not determined solely by weight or diet, but by a constellation of lifestyle factors, including mental health.

Sleep Deprivation: The Overlooked Culprit

Modern society often glorifies productivity at the expense of sleep. Yet, research consistently shows that sleeping fewer than six hours per night significantly increases the risk of type 2 diabetes. Sleep deprivation disrupts hunger hormones, impairs glucose metabolism, and makes healthy choices harder to sustain.

Timeline: The Shift to a Modern Lifestyle

- **Industrial Revolution (late 18th to early 19th centuries):** Introduction of mass-produced foods and urban living reduces physical activity.
- **Mid-20th Century:** Processed foods become commonplace; television and cars promote sedentary habits.
- **Late 20th to Early 21st Century:** Digital technology, urbanization, and globalized food systems accelerate lifestyle changes worldwide.

Key Features of the Modern Lifestyle That Raise Diabetes Risk

- **Reduced physical activity:** Desk jobs and screen-based leisure dominate.
- **Increased consumption of processed foods:** High in sugar, fat, and calories.
- **Chronic stress:** From work, social expectations, and digital overload.
- **Poor sleep patterns:** Short, irregular, or disrupted sleep.
- **Lack of community or social support:** Urban isolation can undermine healthy habits.
- **Exposure to environmental toxins:** From plastics to air pollution, these factors may also play a role in metabolic health.

Modern Lifestyle Impacts Metabolic Health

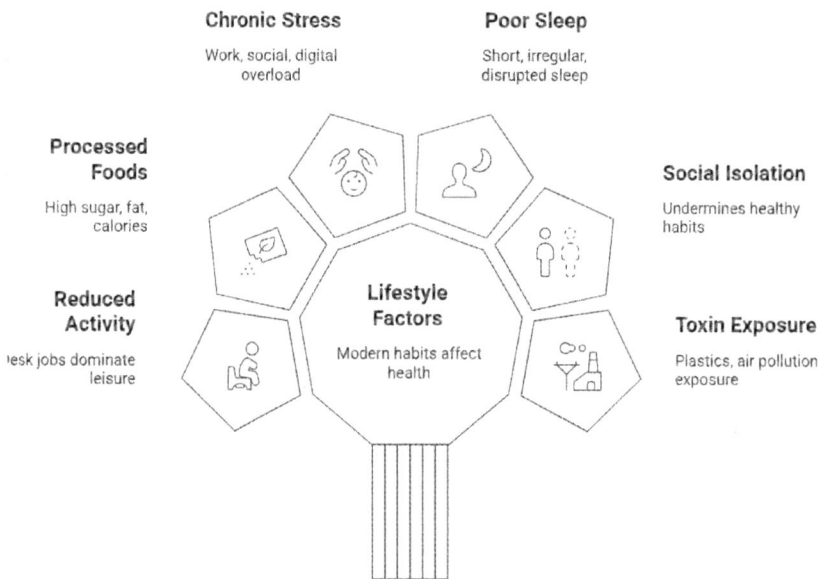

A Global Perspective

Although the narrative of modernization is often associated with Western countries, the diabetes crisis has become truly global. In urban China, for example, rates of type 2 diabetes have quadrupled in the past 30 years as lifestyles shift away from traditional, plant-based diets and daily movement. Meanwhile, Indigenous populations in Australia and North America, whose ancestors thrived on natural, unprocessed foods, now face some of the world's highest rates of diabetes after adopting modern dietary and lifestyle patterns.

What This Means for You

The modern lifestyle is not our destiny—it's a context we can navigate. By recognizing the forces at play, we become equipped to make choices that counteract the risks embedded in our environment.

```
- Fact: Sitting for more than 8 hours a day without physical activity can
increase the risk of developing type 2 diabetes by up to 90%.
- Important: Chronic stress raises blood sugar even in the absence of poor
diet or inactivity.
```

2.3 The Role of Obesity

Obesity stands as one of the most significant and modifiable risk factors for type 2 diabetes. Its impact stretches beyond aesthetics or body size, touching the very core of how our bodies process energy, regulate hormones, and respond to the food we eat. Understanding the intricate relationship between excess weight and diabetes provides not just clarity, but hope—because unlike genetics or age, this is a risk factor we can change.

How Obesity Fuels Type 2 Diabetes

The link between obesity and type 2 diabetes is both direct and multi-layered. At its heart lies the concept of **insulin resistance**. In those carrying excess weight—especially around the abdomen—fat cells produce inflammatory substances and hormones that interfere with the body's ability to use insulin effectively. The pancreas compensates by working overtime to produce even more insulin. Over time, this system begins to falter, leading to higher blood sugar levels and, eventually, the diagnosis of type 2 diabetes.

But why does fat have such a powerful effect on insulin? The answer lies in the type of fat and its location in the body.

- **Visceral fat** (fat stored deep within the abdomen) is particularly harmful. It wraps around internal organs and is metabolically active, releasing substances that can disrupt normal metabolic function.
- **Subcutaneous fat** (the fat just under the skin) has a less pronounced effect but still contributes to overall insulin resistance over time.

A Global Epidemic

Obesity and type 2 diabetes are not challenges unique to any one country or culture—they are truly global in scale. While the Western world has grappled with rising waistlines for decades, countries undergoing rapid economic change are seeing the same trend emerge—often at an even faster pace.

Consider the story of **Mexico**, a nation that, in just a single generation, has seen a dramatic rise in both obesity and diabetes rates. Traditional diets rich in beans, vegetables, and whole grains have been replaced by processed foods high in sugars and unhealthy fats. As a result, Mexico now has one of the highest rates of diabetes in the world. Families that once thrived on homemade, balanced meals are now facing an epidemic of chronic disease—an urgent reminder of how quickly environment and lifestyle can reshape health.

In contrast, **Japan** provides an illuminating example of how cultural habits can protect against, or contribute to, obesity-related diabetes. For much of the 20th century, Japan's diet was based on fish, rice, and vegetables, with minimal processed food. Diabetes rates were low. However, as Western-style fast food became more common, so did obesity and type 2 diabetes, especially among the younger generation. These two stories illustrate that while genetics play a role, environment and lifestyle are potent forces in either fueling or fighting this disease.

The Timeline: Obesity and Disease Progression

The relationship between weight gain and diabetes typically unfolds in a predictable pattern:

- **Weight Gain**: Often gradual, sometimes accelerating during periods of stress, inactivity, or dietary change.
- **Insulin Resistance**: As excess fat accumulates, particularly in the abdomen, the body's cells become less responsive to insulin.
- **Compensatory Hyperinsulinemia**: The pancreas produces more insulin in an attempt to keep blood sugar in check.
- **Pancreatic Fatigue**: Over time, the pancreas becomes unable to keep up with demand.
- **Rising Blood Sugar**: Blood sugar levels increase, leading to prediabetes and, unless reversed, type 2 diabetes.

Key Takeaways

Obesity is a primary, modifiable risk factor for type 2 diabetes.

Visceral fat is particularly harmful due to its effect on insulin resistance.

Cultural and environmental changes can dramatically influence rates of obesity and diabetes.

Fact: Losing just 5-7% of your body weight can reduce the risk of developing type 2 diabetes by more than 50% in high-risk individuals.

Reflecting on What We Can Change

Obesity's role in type 2 diabetes is both sobering and empowering. While the global rise in obesity threatens public health on a massive scale, it also presents a unique opportunity for positive change. By understanding the mechanisms at play and sharing real stories of transformation, we can inspire actionable hope.

As we transition into the next section, we'll dive deeper into how dietary choices shape our risk—and how, meal by meal, we can reclaim control over our health and future.

2.4 Stress and Sleep

Stress and sleep are two often-overlooked but profoundly influential factors in the development and progression of type 2 diabetes. While genetics, diet, and physical activity are widely recognized contributors, the intricate interplay between emotional well-being, rest, and metabolic health is only now gaining the full attention it deserves. Understanding how chronic stress and inadequate sleep act as silent saboteurs can empower us to make meaningful changes—restoring balance not just to our blood sugar, but to our entire lives.

The Physiology of Stress: When Fight or Flight Goes Awry

The human stress response, honed over millennia, was designed for survival. When our ancestors faced threats—a prowling predator, a sudden storm—the **fight-or-flight** response flooded their bodies with hormones like cortisol and adrenaline. Blood sugar surged to fuel muscles, preparing for action.

In the modern world, the threats we face are rarely physical. Deadlines, financial worries, and family responsibilities activate the same physiological pathways. Chronically elevated stress hormones now serve no productive purpose. Instead, they wreak havoc on our metabolism.

> **Cortisol**, the primary stress hormone, signals the liver to release more glucose into the bloodstream.
> Persistent high cortisol levels can lead to **insulin resistance**, making it harder for cells to absorb glucose.
> Stress often triggers unhealthy coping mechanisms—overeating, alcohol use, or inactivity—that further disrupt blood sugar control.

A compelling example comes from a study of Japanese "karoshi" (death from overwork) cases. In the 1980s and 1990s, researchers noted a sharp increase in diabetes and cardiovascular deaths among workers enduring chronic, unrelenting stress and long hours. This tragic phenomenon underscores how prolonged psychological strain can manifest as physical disease.

The Power of Restorative Sleep

Just as stress disrupts, sleep restores. Yet, in our fast-paced world, sleep is often sacrificed for productivity or entertainment. For those at risk of, or living with, type 2 diabetes, this is a dangerous trade-off.

Sleep is when the body repairs itself, resets hormonal balances, and consolidates memories—including those related to healthy habits. But sleep deprivation or poor sleep quality can quickly undermine these benefits:

- **Short sleep duration** (less than 6 hours per night) is associated with higher blood sugar levels and increased risk of developing type 2 diabetes.
- **Disrupted sleep**—such as from sleep apnea or frequent nighttime awakenings—raises stress hormones, increasing insulin resistance.
- **Lack of sleep** often leads to increased appetite for high-calorie, high-sugar foods, further compounding metabolic risk.

One vivid example is the Pima people of the American Southwest, who have some of the highest rates of type 2 diabetes in the world. Researchers found that Pima individuals who reported the least sleep had the greatest difficulty managing blood sugar, regardless of their diet or physical activity. This finding, echoed globally, highlights the universal importance of sleep in diabetes prevention and reversal.

Breaking the Cycle: Stress, Sleep, and Self-Care

The relationship between stress, sleep, and type 2 diabetes can become a vicious cycle. Stress leads to poor sleep; poor sleep increases stress. Both undermine metabolic health, making lifestyle changes feel overwhelming. Recognizing this cycle is the first step to breaking it.

Consider the story of Priya, a London-based accountant. After her type 2 diabetes diagnosis, she focused solely on diet and medication, frustrated by slow progress. It wasn't until a diabetes educator suggested mindfulness meditation and a consistent bedtime routine that things changed. Within weeks, Priya reported better sleep, less emotional eating, and improved blood sugar readings. Her experience, echoed by countless others, highlights the transformative power of addressing stress and sleep.

Practical Strategies for Lasting Change

Making stress reduction and quality sleep central to your diabetes management does not require drastic measures, but it does require conscious effort:

Strategies for Diabetes Management

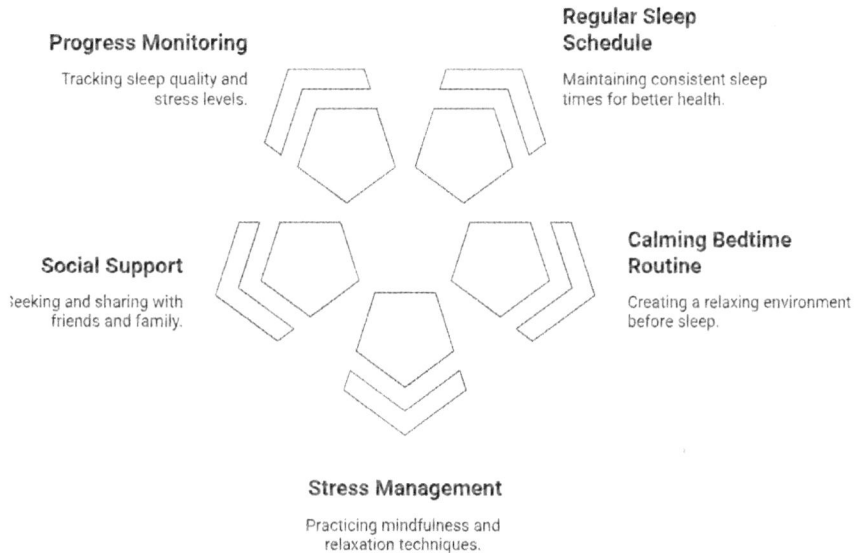

Progress Monitoring

Tracking sleep quality and stress levels.

Regular Sleep Schedule

Maintaining consistent sleep times for better health.

Social Support

Seeking and sharing with friends and family.

Calming Bedtime Routine

Creating a relaxing environment before sleep.

Stress Management

Practicing mindfulness and relaxation techniques.

- **Establish a regular sleep schedule**—Go to bed and wake up at the same time daily, even on weekends.
- **Create a calming bedtime routine**—Limit screens, dim the lights, and engage in relaxing activities before bed.
- **Practice stress management**—Explore mindfulness, deep breathing, or gentle yoga. Even 5-10 minutes daily can make a difference.
- **Seek support**—Share your challenges with friends, family, or a counselor. Social connection is a powerful buffer against stress.
- **Monitor progress**—Keep a journal to track sleep quality, stress levels, and how you feel physically and emotionally.

A Global Perspective: Cultural Views on Stress and Sleep

Around the world, different cultures approach stress and sleep in unique ways. In Scandinavian countries, for example, the concept of "hygge" emphasizes coziness, relaxation, and social connection—values linked to lower stress and better sleep. In contrast, the high-pressure environments of some East Asian cities reveal the health costs of chronic stress and sleep deprivation, as seen in the karoshi phenomenon.

By drawing from diverse traditions—whether it's the afternoon siesta in Spain or the evening tea ritual in Morocco—anyone can cultivate healthier rhythms that support diabetes reversal.

Chronic stress and poor sleep are powerful, modifiable risk factors for type 2 diabetes—addressing them can significantly improve your odds of prevention and reversal.

2.5 Societal Influences

Over the past several decades, the landscape of type 2 diabetes has shifted dramatically—not just due to changes in individual habits, but also as a result of powerful societal forces at play. To truly understand how type 2 diabetes has become a global epidemic, it's essential to look beyond personal choices and examine the broader context in which those choices are made. From the convenience-driven evolution of our food systems to the digital transformation of our daily lives, societal influences shape our health in profound and often subtle ways.

The Rise of Processed Foods and Fast Food Culture

One of the most significant societal shifts contributing to the diabetes epidemic is the proliferation of highly processed, calorie-dense foods. In the mid-20th century, the advent of industrial food processing brought about an explosion of packaged snacks, sugary beverages, and ready-to-eat meals. These products were marketed as modern, convenient solutions for busy families, quickly becoming staples in kitchens worldwide.

Causes of the Diabetes Epidemic

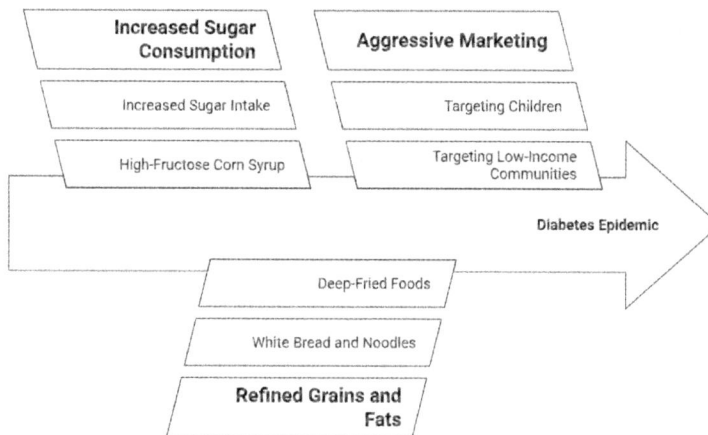

- **Increased Sugar Consumption:** The average global sugar intake has more than doubled in the last 50 years. In the United States, for example, the introduction of high-fructose corn syrup in the 1970s made sweetened beverages and snacks more accessible and affordable.

- **Refined Grains and Fats:** White bread, instant noodles, and deep-fried foods replaced traditional whole grains and home-cooked meals in many cultures, leading to increased blood sugar spikes and insulin resistance.
- **Aggressive Marketing:** Food companies have targeted children and low-income communities, making processed foods the easy, affordable choice.

Real-World Example: In Mexico, the spread of Western-style fast food and sugary sodas has paralleled a sharp rise in type 2 diabetes rates. Today, Mexico is among the top consumers of soda per capita, and diabetes is now a leading cause of death in the country.

Sedentary Lifestyles in a Digital Age

Modern technology, while improving many aspects of life, has also contributed to a dramatic reduction in physical activity. The transition from labor-intensive jobs and active transportation to desk work, screen time, and motorized transport has made sedentary behavior the norm.

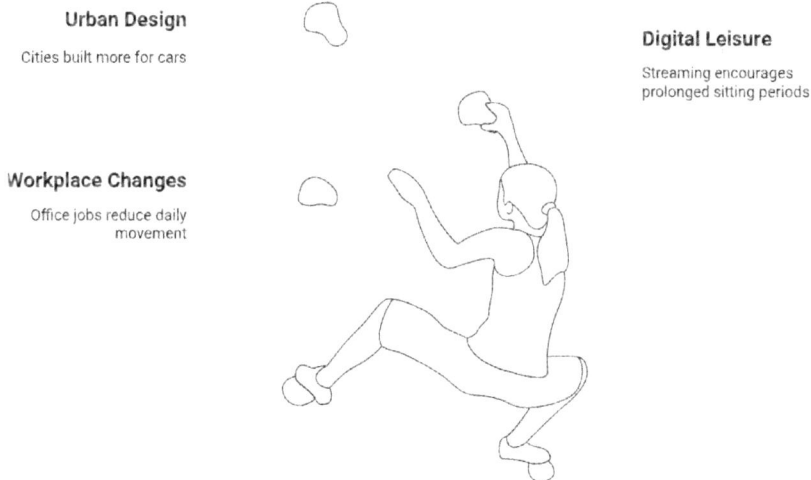

Sedentary Lifestyles: A Modern Crisis

Urban Design
Cities built more for cars

Digital Leisure
Streaming encourages prolonged sitting periods

Workplace Changes
Office jobs reduce daily movement

- **Workplace Changes:** The rise of office jobs and remote work has cut down on daily movement. Walking to work or engaging in manual labor is less common than in previous generations.

- **Digital Leisure:** Streaming services, video games, and social media encourage prolonged periods of sitting, displacing time once spent outdoors or engaged in physical play.
- **Urban Design:** Many cities are built for cars, not pedestrians or cyclists, limiting opportunities for incidental exercise.

Personal Story: Maria, a 42-year-old office worker from Manila, recalls her childhood spent playing tag in the streets and eating homemade meals. As her city modernized, her commute lengthened, her work became computer-based, and meals were increasingly sourced from fast-food chains. She was diagnosed with type 2 diabetes at age 39—a story echoed by millions worldwide.

Economic and Social Determinants of Health

Type 2 diabetes does not develop in a vacuum. Economic pressures, cultural norms, and social structures all influence risk factors and health outcomes.

- **Food Deserts:** In many urban and rural areas, especially in low-income communities, fresh fruits and vegetables are scarce or unaffordable, while fast food and convenience stores thrive.
- **Healthcare Access:** Lack of affordable, preventive healthcare and education means diabetes often goes undiagnosed and untreated until complications arise.
- **Cultural Traditions:** Some societies prize large, calorie-rich meals as a symbol of hospitality or prosperity, making portion control and dietary changes challenging.

Historical Anecdote: In the Pacific Islands, traditional diets rich in fish, root vegetables, and fruits kept diabetes rare for centuries. Following World War II, the introduction of imported white rice, canned meats, and sugary drinks—coupled with a decline in physical activity—resulted in a surge of diabetes cases, now among the highest rates in the world.

Globalization and the Spread of Western Lifestyles

The globalization of food supply chains and media has fueled the adoption of Western eating and lifestyle patterns in countries previously protected by traditional ways of living. This shift, sometimes called "nutrition transition," has created a perfect storm for the spread of diabetes.

Homogenized Diets: Local, seasonal foods are increasingly replaced by uniform, processed products.

Changing Aspirations: Western standards of convenience, body image, and success influence individual choices, often at odds with healthful traditions.

```
The World Health Organization estimates that over 420 million people worldwide
now live with diabetes—four times the number in 1980—largely driven by
societal changes in diet and activity patterns.
```

Societal influences—ranging from the foods on supermarket shelves to the way our cities are built—play a pivotal role in shaping the type 2 diabetes epidemic. Recognizing these forces is the first step toward forging a new path. By understanding the context in which we make daily decisions, we become empowered to challenge norms and reclaim our health. As we move forward, let's explore how targeted dietary strategies can help you regain control, meal by meal, on the journey to reversing type 2 diabetes and achieving lasting wellness.

2.6 Assessing Your Personal Risk

For many, the realization that type 2 diabetes is not just a distant threat but a personal concern comes as a wake-up call. Recognizing your own risk is the essential first step towards prevention and, if needed, reversal. Understanding the unique constellation of factors that shape your personal risk profile can empower you to make informed, proactive decisions in your daily life.

The Building Blocks of Risk

Type 2 diabetes develops from a blend of genetic predisposition, lifestyle choices, and environmental factors. While some risk factors are beyond our control, many are modifiable. Let's break down these elements:

- **Family history**: Having a parent or sibling with type 2 diabetes increases your risk significantly.
- **Age**: Risk rises after age 45, but younger adults and even children are increasingly affected due to changing lifestyles.
- **Weight and body fat distribution**: Carrying excess weight, especially around the abdomen, is a major risk factor.
- **Physical inactivity**: Leading a sedentary life slows metabolism and increases insulin resistance.
- **Ethnicity**: Certain populations—including African, South Asian, Hispanic/Latino, Pacific Islander, and Native American communities—face higher risks.
- **History of gestational diabetes**: Women who have had diabetes during pregnancy, or who have given birth to a baby over 9 pounds, are at heightened risk.

- **Polycystic ovary syndrome (PCOS)**: Women with PCOS are more likely to develop type 2 diabetes.

Self-Assessment: Gauging Your Risk

The process of self-assessment is both science and self-reflection. Medical professionals use various scoring systems—such as the American Diabetes Association's Risk Test or the Finnish Diabetes Risk Score (FINDRISC)—to estimate risk. You can also take stock of your personal habits and medical history:

Exploring Type 2 Diabetes Risk Factors

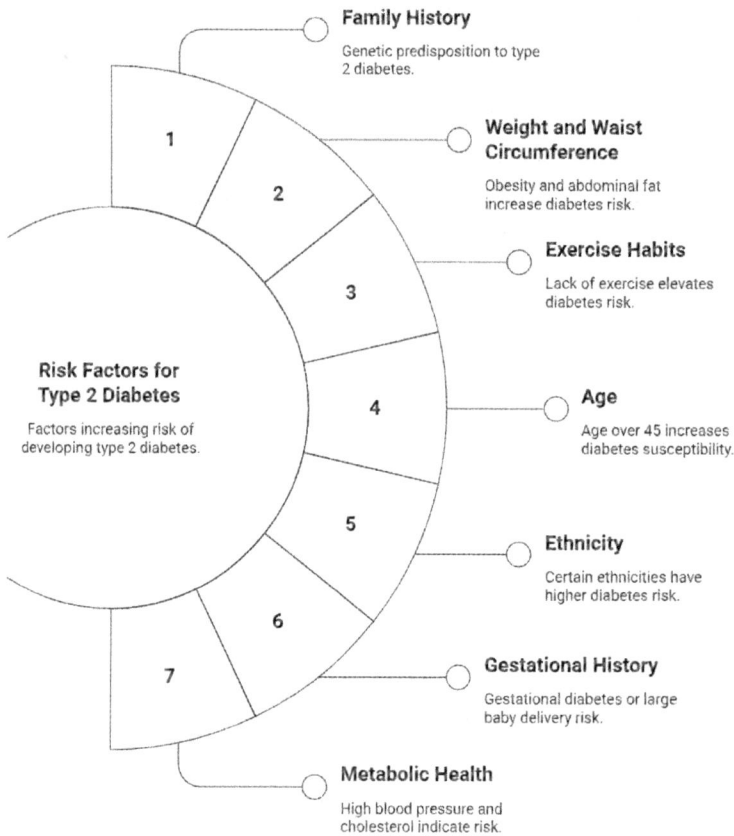

Family History
Genetic predisposition to type 2 diabetes.

Weight and Waist Circumference
Obesity and abdominal fat increase diabetes risk.

Exercise Habits
Lack of exercise elevates diabetes risk.

Age
Age over 45 increases diabetes susceptibility.

Ethnicity
Certain ethnicities have higher diabetes risk.

Gestational History
Gestational diabetes or large baby delivery risk.

Metabolic Health
High blood pressure and cholesterol indicate risk.

Risk Factors for Type 2 Diabetes
Factors increasing risk of developing type 2 diabetes.

Checklist for Self-Evaluation

- Do you have a family member with type 2 diabetes?
- Are you overweight or obese, especially with weight concentrated around your waist?
- Do you exercise less than three times a week?

- Are you over the age of 45?
- Are you from a higher-risk ethnic background?
- Did you have gestational diabetes or deliver a large baby?
- Do you have high blood pressure, high cholesterol, or signs of metabolic syndrome?

If you answered "yes" to several of these questions, it's time to consider yourself at increased risk—and to act accordingly.

Personal Stories: Turning Points and Wake-Up Calls

Sometimes, risk only becomes real through the lens of personal experience. Consider the story of **Anita**, a 38-year-old mother of two from Mumbai. Despite being busy with her career and family, she rarely exercised and often ate takeout meals. Her wake-up call came after a routine health check-up revealed elevated blood sugar levels. With a family history of diabetes, she recognized her risk and chose to overhaul her lifestyle—embracing daily walks, cooking at home, and prioritizing her health. Within six months, her blood sugar normalized, underscoring the power of early recognition and intervention.

On a broader scale, the Pima Indians of Arizona provide a stark historical example. Once reliant on traditional, high-fiber diets and physically active lifestyles, their rates of type 2 diabetes were negligible. However, with the shift to processed foods and a more sedentary lifestyle in the 20th century, diabetes rates soared to among the highest in the world. This story is a sobering reminder that lifestyle shifts can dramatically alter risk—even across generations.

The Silent Progression: Why Early Awareness Matters

Type 2 diabetes often develops quietly, with symptoms that may be subtle or mistaken for everyday fatigue or stress. By the time classic signs—such as excessive thirst, frequent urination, or blurred vision—emerge, the condition may have been present for years. That's why early risk assessment is so crucial.

Pre-diabetes: This is a stage where blood sugar is elevated but not yet in the diabetes range. It's both a warning and an opportunity: lifestyle changes at this point are highly effective in preventing progression.

Global Perspectives: Risk Across Borders

Risk factors are not distributed equally around the globe. Urbanization, dietary changes, and reduced physical activity have led to rising rates of type 2 diabetes in both developed and developing nations. In Japan, for example, traditional diets rich in fish, vegetables, and rice protected previous generations. Yet as Western-style fast food has become more popular, younger urban dwellers are seeing increased rates of diabetes. These global patterns reinforce the importance of environment and culture in shaping our risk.

Action Steps: What You Can Do Today

- Schedule a check-up with your healthcare provider if you have several risk factors.
- Track your waist circumference and weight over time.
- Begin a journal to record your daily activity and eating habits.
- Share your concerns and goals with family members, turning self-care into a shared journey.

Memorable Fact: Most people with pre-diabetes can prevent or delay type 2 diabetes with moderate weight loss (5-7% of body weight) and regular physical activity.
Very Important: Risk assessment is not just about numbers—it's about recognizing opportunities for change before symptoms appear.

Assessing your personal risk isn't about fear—it's about empowerment. By understanding your unique risk profile, you're taking the first, most important step toward lasting health. In the next section, we'll delve deeper into how targeted dietary strategies can help you regain control, meal by meal, on the journey to reversing type 2 diabetes and achieving lasting wellness.

3 : The Turning Point – Diagnosis and Early Intervention

3.1 How Is Type 2 Diabetes Diagnosed?

For many, the path to a type 2 diabetes diagnosis begins not with a single dramatic symptom, but with a subtle accumulation of warning signs—unexplained fatigue, increased thirst, frequent urination, or blurred vision. Some individuals, however, experience no symptoms at all, learning of their condition only through routine health screenings. This variability makes understanding the diagnostic process all the more crucial.

The Diagnostic Steps: Tests That Reveal the Truth

Diagnosing type 2 diabetes is a methodical process grounded in standardized medical tests. These tests measure how well your body manages glucose, the primary sugar circulating in your blood. The following are the most commonly used diagnostic tools:

Diabetes Diagnostic Tests

	Measurement Timing	Measurement Reflected
Fasting Plasma Glucose (FPG)	After overnight fast	Current blood sugar level
Hemoglobin A1c (HbA1c)	No specific timing	Average blood glucose (2-3 months)
Oral Glucose Tolerance (OGTT)	Before and after glucose drink	Body's glucose processing ability
Random Plasma Glucose	Any time	Current blood sugar level

- **Fasting Plasma Glucose (FPG) Test**: Measures blood sugar after an overnight fast.

- **Hemoglobin A1c (HbA1c) Test**: Reflects average blood glucose over the past 2-3 months.
- **Oral Glucose Tolerance Test (OGTT)**: Measures blood sugar before and after consuming a glucose-rich drink.
- **Random Plasma Glucose Test**: Measures blood sugar at any time, regardless of when you last ate.

Each of these tests provides a unique snapshot of blood sugar control. Let's walk through the diagnostic sequence as it typically unfolds:

Routine Screening or Symptom Recognition

- Many diagnoses begin with routine screenings, especially for those at higher risk (e.g., family history, overweight, certain ethnic backgrounds).

- Alternatively, the presence of classic symptoms (excessive thirst, frequent urination, unexplained weight loss) prompts testing.

Initial Blood Sugar Testing

- The doctor orders one or more of the above tests. Fasting plasma glucose and HbA1c are the most common starting points.

- For the FPG test, a result of **126 mg/dL (7.0 mmol/L)** or higher on two separate occasions confirms diabetes.

- For the HbA1c test, a level of **6.5% or higher** is diagnostic.

Confirmation and Further Testing

- If results are borderline or inconsistent, additional tests such as OGTT may be used for clarity.

- The OGTT involves measuring blood sugar two hours after drinking a sweet liquid; a result of **200 mg/dL (11.1 mmol/L)** or higher confirms diabetes.

Diagnosis and Early Intervention

- Once type 2 diabetes is confirmed, the focus shifts to early intervention: education, lifestyle changes, and sometimes medication.

The Global Picture: Diverse Practices and Early Detection

Around the world, approaches to diabetes diagnosis and early intervention reflect a blend of medical protocol and cultural context. In the United States, the **Centers for**

Disease Control and Prevention (CDC) recommends screening adults over 45 and younger people with risk factors. In contrast, some Scandinavian countries have instituted widespread workplace wellness screenings, aiming to catch cases even before symptoms arise.

A historical perspective can be found in the story of **Dr. Elliott Joslin**, a pioneering American diabetologist in the early 20th century. Dr. Joslin emphasized not only the importance of early diagnosis but also the power of patient education, advocating for individuals to take charge of their health—a principle that remains at the heart of diabetes care today.

The Importance of Timely Diagnosis

Early diagnosis of type 2 diabetes is more than just a medical formality—it's a gateway to intervention and, potentially, reversal. Undiagnosed or untreated diabetes can quietly damage the heart, kidneys, nerves, and eyes, often before outward symptoms become severe. The sooner you know, the sooner you can act.

```
Fact: Nearly one in two adults with type 2 diabetes worldwide remain
undiagnosed, increasing the risk of serious complications. Early testing saves
lives.
```

What Happens After Diagnosis?

A diagnosis may feel overwhelming, but it is also empowering. Like Maya, many find that knowing their status brings clarity and motivation. The next steps—education, support, and a tailored action plan—form the foundation for managing and potentially reversing the disease.

As we move forward, the next section will explore the immediate actions you can take after diagnosis—transforming knowledge into practical steps for reclaiming your well-being and setting yourself on the road to reversal.

3.2 Understanding Your Numbers

Receiving a diagnosis of type 2 diabetes can feel like stepping into a world where everyday language is replaced by numbers, charts, and acronyms. Suddenly, terms like **A1C**, **fasting glucose**, and **postprandial blood sugar** become central to your daily life. Yet, understanding these numbers is essential—they are the compass guiding your journey toward reversal and lasting health.

Let's demystify these metrics, exploring what they mean, why they matter, and how you can use them as powerful tools for change.

The Key Numbers: What Do They Mean?

Three core measurements form the foundation of diabetes monitoring. Each tells a different part of your story:

- **Fasting Blood Glucose (FBG):** This measures your blood sugar after an overnight fast (usually 8 hours). It provides a snapshot of how well your body manages glucose without the immediate influence of food.
- **Hemoglobin A1C (HbA1c):** This test reflects your average blood sugar levels over the past two to three months. It's a vital indicator of long-term glucose control.
- **Postprandial Glucose:** Taken 1-2 hours after eating, this reading shows how your body handles sugar from food. Spikes here can reveal hidden issues, even if fasting numbers seem normal.

Each of these numbers offers crucial insights, but together, they create a comprehensive picture of your metabolic health.

Understanding the Ranges

Knowing your numbers is only powerful if you understand what they mean in context. Here's a guide to typical diagnostic ranges:

Diagnostic Ranges Comparison

	Normal	Prediabetes	Diabetes
Fasting Blood Glucose	70–99 mg/dL	100–125 mg/dL	126+ mg/dL
Hemoglobin A1C	Below 5.7%	5.7%–6.4%	6.5%+
Postprandial Glucose	140 mg/dL	N/A	200 mg/dL

Fasting Blood Glucose:

- Normal: 70–99 mg/dL (3.9–5.5 mmol/L)

- Prediabetes: 100–125 mg/dL (5.6–6.9 mmol/L)

- Diabetes: 126 mg/dL (7.0 mmol/L) or higher

Hemoglobin A1C:

- Normal: Below 5.7%

- Prediabetes: 5.7%–6.4%

- Diabetes: 6.5% or higher

Postprandial Glucose:

- Normal: Less than 140 mg/dL (7.8 mmol/L)

- Diabetes: Greater than 200 mg/dL (11.1 mmol/L)

These thresholds are based on recommendations from global organizations such as the **American Diabetes Association** and the **World Health Organization**. However, individual targets may differ depending on your age, health status, and physician's advice.

Why Your Numbers Matter: The Turning Point

For many, seeing a high number for the first time is a defining moment—a call to action. Take the story of **Carlos**, a father of three from Mexico City. When his routine blood test revealed an A1C of 8.2%, the shock was immediate. Carlos recalls, "It was like a warning siren I couldn't ignore." With guidance from his healthcare team, Carlos learned to monitor his numbers closely. Within six months, by changing his diet and walking every day with his children, he brought his A1C down to 6.1%. Carlos's story illustrates the transformative power of understanding and acting on your numbers.

The Story Behind the Numbers: A Brief History

The concept of measuring blood sugar has evolved dramatically. In the early 20th century, people with diabetes had few tools for self-monitoring. It wasn't until the 1970s that home glucose meters became widely available, shifting diabetes care from hospitals to homes. The development of the A1C test in the late 1970s was another watershed moment, providing a reliable way to track long-term glucose control. Today, continuous glucose monitors (CGMs) offer real-time feedback, empowering people to make immediate lifestyle adjustments.

Tracking Your Progress: Building a Personal Timeline

Monitoring your numbers is not a one-time event but an ongoing process. Here's how to create a meaningful timeline:

- **Establish Your Baseline:** Record your initial readings at diagnosis.

- **Set Realistic Goals:** With your healthcare provider, determine target ranges for each metric.
- **Track Regularly:** Use a diary, app, or CGM to log readings and spot trends.
- **Review and Adjust:** Meet with your care team regularly to review progress and tweak your plan.
- **Celebrate Milestones:** Recognize improvements, however small—they're signs of progress and resilience.

Making the Most of Your Numbers: Practical Tips

- **Consistency Is Key:** Test at the same times each day for reliable comparisons.
- **Note Food and Activity:** Write down meals, snacks, and exercise to understand their impact.
- **Share Results:** Bring your log to appointments. Collaboration with your healthcare team is vital.

```
Fact: Lowering your A1C by just 1% can reduce the risk of diabetes-related
complications by up to 40%.
Very Important: Regular monitoring empowers you to catch trends early,
preventing serious health crises.
```

Understanding your numbers is not about judgment; it's about empowerment. Each reading is a data point—an opportunity to make informed decisions and reclaim control over your health. Carlos's story and the broader history of diabetes care remind us: knowledge isn't just power; it's the first step toward transformation.

As we move forward, the next section will translate these insights into concrete actions. You'll learn how to turn your new understanding into daily habits that not only stabilize your numbers but also unlock the possibility of true reversal and lasting health.

3.3 The Critical Window for Change

The period immediately following a **type 2 diabetes diagnosis** is a pivotal juncture—a "critical window" during which the body is often most responsive to positive change. The diagnosis, while daunting, offers a unique chance to intervene before lasting damage occurs or medications become a lifelong necessity. This window is not merely a metaphor; it is grounded in clinical evidence and echoed in the stories of countless individuals who have reclaimed their health.

The Science Behind Early Intervention

When type 2 diabetes is first diagnosed, most people still retain a substantial degree of **insulin sensitivity** and pancreatic function. The body's cells, though resistant, are not yet completely unresponsive to insulin, and the pancreas is still producing some insulin. At this stage:

- Blood sugar levels are elevated, but often not dangerously so.
- Complications like nerve damage, kidney disease, or vision loss are typically minimal or absent.
- Lifestyle interventions—diet, exercise, stress management—are most effective in restoring balance.

Multiple studies confirm that **early intervention** can halt, and in some cases reverse, the trajectory of type 2 diabetes. The famous **Diabetes Prevention Program (DPP)** in the United States, for example, found that people at high risk who made intensive lifestyle changes reduced their risk of developing diabetes by 58%, outperforming medication alone.

What Happens During the Critical Window?

The first weeks and months post-diagnosis are a period of both vulnerability and opportunity. Here's what typically unfolds:

- **Diagnosis:** Blood tests reveal elevated glucose (A1C, fasting glucose), prompting a formal diagnosis.
- **Assessment:** Healthcare providers assess risk factors, existing complications, and readiness for change.
- **Action Plan:** Together, you and your care team outline a personalized strategy, focusing on nutrition, movement, and stress reduction.
- **Implementation:** You begin making tangible changes—altering meals, increasing activity, monitoring blood sugar.
- **Adjustment:** Based on early results, your plan is fine-tuned for optimal progress.

During this window, even **modest weight loss** (5–10% of body weight) can dramatically improve insulin sensitivity. Dietary shifts—especially reducing high-glycemic foods—can quickly lower blood sugar. Physical activity acts as a catalyst, drawing glucose out of the bloodstream and improving how your body uses insulin.

The Global Perspective: Opportunities and Obstacles

Globally, the critical window may look different depending on cultural, economic, and healthcare realities. In Japan, for instance, government-sponsored health screenings catch diabetes early for millions, allowing for swift intervention. In contrast, in parts of sub-Saharan Africa, limited access to screening means many people are diagnosed late, after complications have set in.

What unites these diverse contexts is the principle that **early recognition and action**—supported by family, community, and health systems—yields the best outcomes.

Overcoming Psychological Barriers

The emotional impact of diagnosis is profound. Denial, fear, or overwhelm can stall action during this window. However, reframing the diagnosis as an opportunity for empowerment, rather than a life sentence, can help unlock motivation.

- **Seek support:** Connecting with others—friends, family, or support groups—can provide accountability and encouragement.
- **Celebrate small wins:** Every healthy meal or walk counts toward a bigger goal.
- **Focus on what you gain:** Improved energy, mood, and long-term health are powerful motivators.

```
- The first 6-12 months after a type 2 diabetes diagnosis is when lifestyle
changes are most likely to reverse the disease's course.
- Early action can help some people reduce or even eliminate the need for
medication.
```

The critical window for change is a fleeting but powerful opportunity. Taking decisive, informed action soon after diagnosis gives you the best odds for reversal and lasting health. As we move forward, we'll explore the practical strategies—starting with dietary changes—that can help you capitalize on this window and reshape your future.

3.4 Emotional Impact of Diagnosis

The moment a diagnosis of type 2 diabetes is delivered often serves as a profound turning point—one that is as psychological as it is physical. For many, hearing the words "You have type 2 diabetes" is not just a medical statement; it reverberates through every aspect of their identity, routines, and relationships. This emotional impact can shape the choices people make in the critical days and weeks that follow, ultimately influencing their ability to reverse the condition and regain their health.

The Emotional Rollercoaster

A diagnosis frequently triggers a cascade of emotions. Some people experience immediate shock or disbelief, particularly if they felt few symptoms or believed themselves healthy. Others feel fear, anger, or guilt—wondering if their past food choices, lifestyle habits, or family history are to blame.

- **Shock and Denial:** Many initially struggle to accept the diagnosis, especially if they lack obvious symptoms. This denial can delay crucial early interventions.
- **Fear and Anxiety:** Concerns about long-term complications—such as vision loss, heart disease, or amputation—can be overwhelming. The fear of dependency on medication or insulin injections looms large.
- **Guilt and Shame:** Some blame themselves, internalizing the diagnosis as a personal failure rather than a complex interplay of genetic and environmental influences.
- **Anger and Frustration:** There can be frustration at the perceived unfairness of the diagnosis or anger directed at healthcare systems, family, or even themselves.

These emotional responses are not unique to any one culture or background. Across continents, the psychological toll of a chronic diagnosis echoes in diverse but universally human ways.

The Stigma of Diabetes: A Global Perspective

Diabetes carries a unique stigma in many communities. In some parts of India and China, for example, there is a cultural tendency to associate chronic illness with personal weakness or moral failure. This can discourage people from seeking help, discussing their diagnosis, or connecting with support networks. In contrast, some Scandinavian countries have made significant strides in destigmatizing diabetes, emphasizing community support, open discussion, and shared responsibility for health outcomes.

The Importance of Emotional Support

Research consistently shows that emotional well-being is closely linked to diabetes outcomes. Those who receive psychological support—whether from family, friends, peer groups, or mental health professionals—are more likely to adopt and sustain the lifestyle changes necessary for reversal.

Key sources of support include:

- **Family and Friends:** Encouragement, shared meals, and joint exercise routines can foster a sense of togetherness and accountability.
- **Peer Support Groups:** Sharing experiences and strategies reduces isolation and builds motivation.

- **Professional Counseling:** Therapists specializing in chronic illness can help individuals process grief, anxiety, or trauma associated with the diagnosis.

Turning Emotions Into Motivation

Early intervention is most successful when emotional responses are acknowledged and addressed. By transforming fear into determination, and shame into self-compassion, people can harness their emotions as powerful motivators for change.

- **Recognition:** Acknowledge and name the emotions you're experiencing.
- **Connection:** Reach out to others—loved ones, health professionals, or peers—who can provide empathy and guidance.
- **Action:** Set small, achievable goals that build confidence and a sense of progress.

People who receive emotional support after a type 2 diabetes diagnosis are significantly more likely to achieve and maintain blood sugar control—and even remission—compared to those who go it alone.

The emotional impact of a type 2 diabetes diagnosis is profound, shaping the path to reversal as much as any diet or medication. Recognizing and addressing these emotions can transform a moment of crisis into a powerful turning point—a catalyst for lasting health. As we move forward, we'll explore the practical dietary strategies that, when combined with emotional resilience, form the foundation for reversing type 2 diabetes and reclaiming your well-being.

3.5 Building a Healthcare Team

A diagnosis of type 2 diabetes is often a watershed moment—a signal that life's routines and priorities must change. In the initial haze of shock, fear, and confusion, many people find themselves overwhelmed by questions: What does this mean for my future? Where do I begin? It is at this critical turning point that assembling a **healthcare team** becomes not just helpful, but essential. Managing and potentially reversing type 2 diabetes is a journey best undertaken with knowledgeable guides and compassionate allies.

Who Should Be on Your Team?

A well-rounded healthcare team brings together a spectrum of expertise. Each professional plays a unique role, contributing to a holistic approach to diabetes management. Your team may include:

Healthcare Team Roles

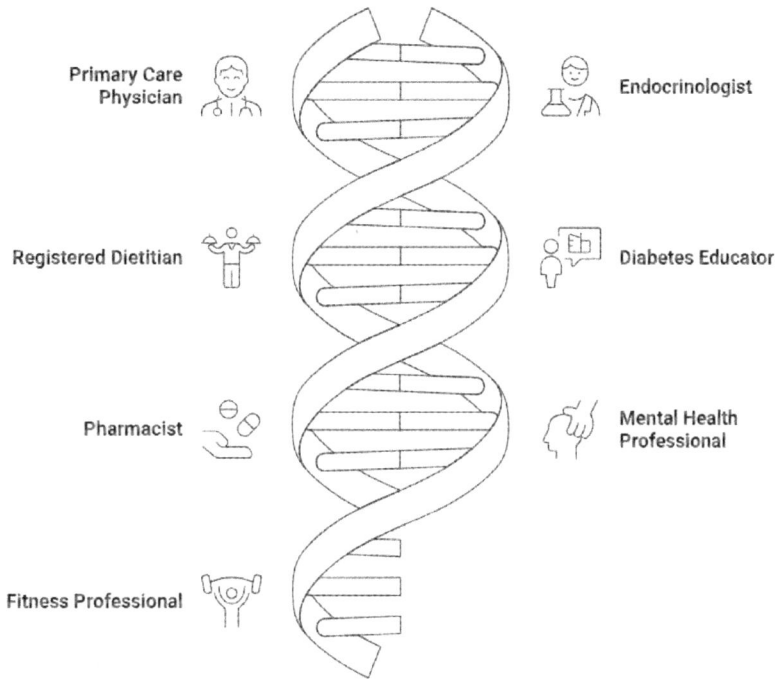

- **Primary Care Physician (PCP):** The central coordinator of your care, responsible for monitoring your overall health, ordering lab tests, adjusting medications, and making referrals.
- **Endocrinologist:** A specialist in hormonal disorders, including diabetes, who can provide advanced guidance if blood sugar control proves challenging.
- **Registered Dietitian (RD) or Nutritionist:** An expert in translating nutritional science into practical meal plans tailored to your specific needs, including glycemic index management and cultural preferences.
- **Certified Diabetes Care and Education Specialist (CDCES):** A professional skilled in diabetes self-management education, offering advice on blood glucose monitoring, medication use, and lifestyle adjustments.
- **Pharmacist:** A valuable resource for understanding medications, potential side effects, and interactions.
- **Mental Health Professional:** Someone to help navigate the psychological impact of diagnosis, address anxiety or depression, and build resilience.
- **Fitness Professional or Physical Therapist:** An ally in developing a safe, effective exercise routine that respects your current abilities and goals.

Real-World Story: Maria's Team Approach

Consider the story of **Maria Alvarez**, a 47-year-old teacher from Texas, who was diagnosed with type 2 diabetes after a routine check-up. Overwhelmed, Maria initially focused only on medication. But her primary care physician encouraged her to meet with a diabetes educator and a registered dietitian. The educator taught her how to monitor her blood sugar, while the dietitian walked her through meal planning that respected her Mexican heritage—incorporating familiar foods like beans and squash, but with a keen eye on glycemic load. With the support of her team, Maria also began working with a physical therapist to safely increase her activity level. Within six months, Maria's blood sugar had improved so much that her doctor was able to reduce her medication.

Maria's story is a testament to the power of a multi-disciplinary approach. Each team member addressed a different aspect of her care, but together, they formed a net of support that made real, sustainable change possible.

Historical Perspective: The Evolution of Team-Based Diabetes Care

Historically, diabetes management was often a solitary affair. In the early 20th century, before the discovery of insulin, treatment options were limited and outcomes were poor. Even after insulin became available, care was typically led by a single physician, with little input from other disciplines. It wasn't until the late 20th century—when research began to reveal the complex interplay of diet, exercise, medication, and psychological health—that the concept of a **multidisciplinary care team** gained traction.

In countries like Sweden, team-based diabetes clinics became models for effective chronic disease management, emphasizing patient education, dietary counseling, and routine follow-up. Today, the World Health Organization recognizes comprehensive, team-based care as a cornerstone of successful diabetes management worldwide.

How to Build and Communicate With Your Team

- **Begin with Your Primary Care Provider:** They can help identify which specialists are most relevant to your situation and make referrals as needed.
- **Be an Active Participant:** Bring questions and concerns to every appointment. Don't hesitate to share challenges—whether they're emotional, practical, or cultural.
- **Coordinate Communication:** Ask for summaries of each visit and share them with other team members to ensure everyone is informed and aligned.

- **Leverage Community Resources:** Many communities offer diabetes support groups, cultural liaisons, or peer mentors who can provide additional guidance and encouragement.

Global Perspectives: Respecting Culture and Context

In India, where vegetarian diets are common, diabetes educators often work closely with local dietitians to craft plant-based meal plans that respect tradition while optimizing blood sugar control. In Australia, Aboriginal health workers play a pivotal role in bridging cultural gaps, ensuring that diabetes care is accessible and relevant to Indigenous communities. These global examples highlight the importance of culturally sensitive care—your healthcare team should respect your background, values, and foodways, making the journey to health both effective and meaningful.

```
- Studies consistently show that people with type 2 diabetes who engage with a
multidisciplinary healthcare team achieve better blood sugar control and are
more likely to reduce or eliminate medication.
- Open communication and cultural sensitivity are crucial for long-term
diabetes management success.
```

Building your healthcare team is not just about assembling experts; it's about creating a circle of support that empowers you to take charge of your health. As you move forward, remember that you are the most important member of this team—your motivation, questions, and daily choices drive the process of reversing type 2 diabetes. In the next section, we'll delve into the heart of diabetes reversal: understanding the power of food and how practical dietary changes can transform your health from the inside out.

3.6 Setting Goals for Health

A type 2 diabetes diagnosis can feel like an abrupt detour on the road of life—disorienting, sometimes frightening, and always significant. But in this moment of uncertainty lies extraordinary opportunity. Setting clear, achievable health goals is the first step toward reclaiming control and initiating meaningful change. These goals serve as a compass, guiding each daily decision toward a healthier future.

The Power of Purposeful Goals

Setting goals is more than ticking boxes; it's about cultivating a sense of purpose and motivation. Research in behavioral psychology shows that individuals who establish concrete, actionable objectives are more likely to make lasting lifestyle changes. When managing or reversing type 2 diabetes, well-defined goals create a roadmap: they break down a daunting journey into manageable steps, making progress visible and setbacks less discouraging.

Consider the story of **Carlos**, a 54-year-old engineer in Mexico City. When diagnosed with type 2 diabetes, Carlos felt overwhelmed by conflicting advice and a flood of new routines. Instead of attempting to overhaul his entire life overnight, he set three specific goals with his doctor: reduce his daily sugar intake by half, walk 30 minutes five days a week, and monitor his blood glucose each morning. Within three months, Carlos saw steady improvement in his blood sugar—and, more importantly, his confidence.

Crafting SMART Goals

The most effective health goals are **SMART**: Specific, Measurable, Achievable, Relevant, and Time-bound. This framework ensures clarity and accountability, transforming vague intentions into tangible action.

Specific: Define exactly what you want to achieve ("I will walk after dinner for 20 minutes" instead of "I should exercise more").

Measurable: Track your progress with numbers ("I will lose 5 pounds in three months").

Achievable: Set realistic targets that challenge you, but are within reach given your current circumstances.

Relevant: Align your goals with your personal values and health needs.

Time-bound: Set deadlines to foster urgency and focus.

Building a Personal Health Timeline

Early intervention is the most powerful weapon against type 2 diabetes progression. Establishing a timeline can help you visualize your journey and anticipate milestones. Here's a simple sequence to get started:

Week 1–2: Assessment and Awareness

- Begin tracking daily food intake and activity levels.

- Schedule a consultation with your healthcare provider.

- Learn your baseline metrics: blood sugar, weight, blood pressure.

Week 3–4: Small, Sustainable Changes

- Identify one dietary habit to modify (swapping sugary beverages for water).

- Introduce light physical activity, like walking or gentle stretching.

- Set up a support system—friends, family, or a diabetes group.

Month 2–3: Building Momentum

- Add another health goal, such as cooking one homemade meal daily.

- Increase physical activity intensity or duration.

- Celebrate progress, no matter how small.

Ongoing: Review and Refine

- Reassess your goals monthly.

- Adjust strategies as needed with your healthcare team's input.

- Keep a journal of setbacks and successes to stay motivated.

Diabetes Management Journey

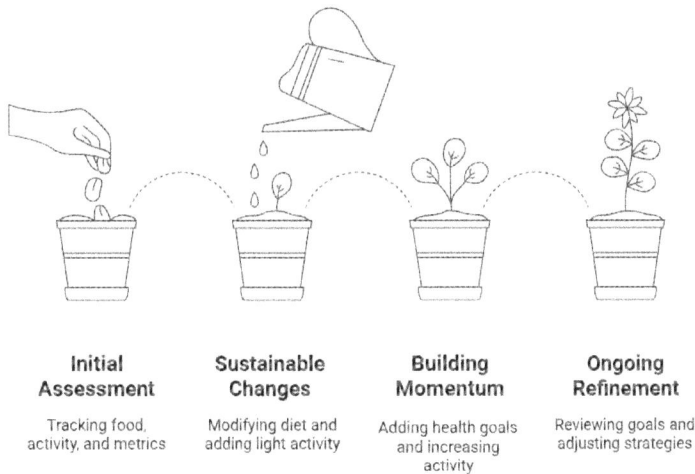

Initial Assessment	Sustainable Changes	Building Momentum	Ongoing Refinement
Tracking food, activity, and metrics	Modifying diet and adding light activity	Adding health goals and increasing activity	Reviewing goals and adjusting strategies

Global Perspectives on Goal-Setting

Approaches to setting health goals vary across cultures, shaped by collective values and societal norms. In Japan, for example, the concept of **kaizen**—continuous, incremental improvement—guides diabetes management. Many Japanese clinics encourage patients to adopt tiny, daily changes, such as adding vegetables to a meal or taking the stairs, fostering a culture of sustainable progress.

Similarly, in South Africa, community-based support plays a vital role. Local diabetes clubs in Cape Town provide not only education but also a network of accountability and encouragement. Members often set shared goals, like participating in group walks or cooking traditional meals with healthier ingredients, blending cultural practices with medical advice.

Overcoming Obstacles

The path to reversing type 2 diabetes is rarely linear. Challenges—stress, social gatherings, travel, or even fatigue—can derail progress. Anticipating setbacks and preparing strategies to address them is crucial. Reflect on past experiences: What has helped you stay committed to a goal before? How can you adapt those strategies to your diabetes journey?

- Lean on support systems during tough times.
- Reframe setbacks as learning opportunities rather than failures.
- Celebrate small wins to reinforce positive behavior.

- Achieving a modest weight loss of 5-10% can significantly improve blood sugar control and reduce medication dependency in many people with type 2 diabetes.
- People who set and regularly review their health goals are up to twice as likely to achieve lasting lifestyle changes compared to those who don't.

Establishing purposeful, achievable goals transforms a diagnosis from a crisis into a catalyst for growth. Whether you find inspiration in Carlos's story, the principle of kaizen, or the strength of community, remember: every small step counts. As you clarify your personal health objectives, you lay the groundwork for lasting change.

In the next section, we'll explore how the foods you choose can further empower you on this journey—unlocking the science of nutrition as a powerful tool for diabetes reversal and lifelong wellness.

4 : The Science of Reversal – Can Type 2 Diabetes Be Reversed?

4.1 Defining Diabetes Reversal and Remission

As we journey deeper into the science underpinning type 2 diabetes reversal, it becomes essential to clarify what "reversal" and "remission" truly mean. These terms are often used interchangeably in everyday conversation, yet they have distinct implications within medical science and for individuals striving to reclaim their health. Defining these concepts is the cornerstone for understanding the possibilities and boundaries of diabetes management, setting realistic expectations, and shaping a path forward that is both hopeful and grounded in evidence.

Understanding Diabetes Reversal

Reversal of type 2 diabetes is a term that stirs hope, yet it should be approached with clarity. In medical parlance, reversal typically refers to the process by which a person with type 2 diabetes achieves normal blood glucose levels without the need for diabetes medications, particularly those that lower blood sugar such as insulin or oral hypoglycemics. However, this does not mean the disease is "cured"—rather, it is under control, and the underlying metabolic vulnerabilities remain.

> **Diabetes reversal** is achieved when blood sugar levels return to non-diabetic ranges (usually a hemoglobin A1c below 6.5%) without medication.
> It is often the result of significant lifestyle changes—especially in diet and physical activity.
> The risk for recurrence remains if old habits return or weight is regained.

The idea of reversal gained traction in the early 21st century, notably with research such as the Newcastle studies in the United Kingdom. In these studies, participants with recently diagnosed type 2 diabetes followed a very low-calorie diet under medical supervision and, in many cases, achieved normal blood sugar levels—sometimes for months or years.

Exploring Remission: A Closer Look

Remission is the term favored by many healthcare professionals and diabetes organizations, including the American Diabetes Association (ADA). It acknowledges both the success of maintaining healthy blood glucose without medication and the chronic, relapsing nature of type 2 diabetes.

Partial remission means blood sugar levels are below the diagnostic threshold for diabetes (A1c < 6.5%) for at least one year without medication, but not necessarily within normal, non-diabetic ranges.

Complete remission is defined as maintaining normal blood sugar levels (A1c in the normal range) for at least one year without medication.

Prolonged remission refers to sustaining this state for five years or longer.

While remission can be achieved, particularly soon after diagnosis, it requires ongoing vigilance and lifestyle maintenance.

Why the Distinction Matters

Understanding the difference between reversal and remission is more than semantic—it shapes how individuals relate to their health and manage their expectations. Reversal implies a return to a previous, disease-free state, while remission acknowledges that the condition is controlled but could recur.

- **Empowerment vs. Complacency:** Some experts caution that the term "reversal" might lead to complacency, as people may believe they are "cured" and can revert to previous habits.
- **Sustained Change:** Remission emphasizes the importance of ongoing lifestyle changes and regular monitoring, even in the absence of symptoms or medication.

Real-World Example: The Story of Maria

Consider the story of **Maria**, a 46-year-old teacher from Mexico City. Diagnosed with type 2 diabetes after years of sedentary living and high-sugar diets, Maria embarked on a comprehensive lifestyle overhaul. She began daily walks in Chapultepec Park, reduced her intake of refined carbohydrates, and embraced traditional Mexican dishes rich in beans, vegetables, and whole grains. Within eight months, her A1c dropped to 5.8%—below the diabetes threshold—and she no longer required medication. Maria's journey exemplifies remission rather than cure: while her diabetes is under control, she continues her healthy habits to maintain these gains.

The Timeline of Reversal and Remission

- **Diagnosis:** Type 2 diabetes is identified, often after years of rising blood sugar.
- **Intervention:** Intensive lifestyle changes—diet, exercise, weight loss—are implemented.
- **Medication Reduction:** As blood sugar normalizes, the need for medication decreases.

- **Remission Achieved:** If normal blood glucose is sustained without medication for at least a year, remission is declared.
- **Maintenance:** Ongoing monitoring and lifestyle adherence are crucial to sustain remission and prevent relapse.

Key Points to Remember

- Reversal is possible, especially for those recently diagnosed and who can make significant lifestyle changes.
- Remission does not mean cure; vigilance and sustained healthy habits are essential.
- Both concepts offer hope and motivation, but also require practical, long-term commitment.

Fact: The earlier type 2 diabetes is addressed with lifestyle changes, the greater the chance for remission—especially within the first 6 years after diagnosis.

Defining reversal and remission sets the stage for understanding what is scientifically possible—and what is required—in the journey to lasting health. These distinctions empower individuals to set realistic goals and inspire sustainable change. In the next section, we will unravel the physiological mechanisms behind reversal, exploring how weight loss, cellular changes, and metabolic flexibility play pivotal roles in reclaiming health.

4.2 Evidence from Research

Over the past two decades, mounting scientific evidence has challenged the belief that type 2 diabetes is an inevitably progressive disease. Instead, researchers have begun to document cases—sometimes in large numbers—where individuals no longer meet the criteria for diabetes after significant lifestyle changes. Among the most influential studies is the **DiRECT trial (Diabetes Remission Clinical Trial)**, conducted in the United Kingdom. Launched in 2014 and published in 2017, DiRECT enrolled over 300 people with recently diagnosed type 2 diabetes. Participants underwent a structured, calorie-restricted diet, followed by gradual food reintroduction and ongoing weight management support.

The results were striking:

- Nearly half of participants (46%) achieved diabetes remission after one year.

- The likelihood of reversal increased with the amount of weight lost: over 80% of those who lost 15 kg (about 33 pounds) or more saw their diabetes go into remission.
- Remission rates were higher among those with a shorter duration of diabetes diagnosis, emphasizing the importance of early intervention.

This study, and others like it, have made it clear: **type 2 diabetes can be reversed in many cases, especially if addressed early and with significant lifestyle change**.

The Role of Bariatric Surgery

Prior to the wave of lifestyle intervention research, a different kind of evidence emerged from the world of bariatric (weight-loss) surgery. In the late 20th and early 21st centuries, doctors noticed that some people with type 2 diabetes who underwent procedures such as **gastric bypass** experienced rapid normalization of blood sugar—even before losing significant weight. This phenomenon suggested that dramatic dietary and anatomical changes could restore the body's ability to regulate glucose.

Though not a solution for everyone, these findings prompted a deeper look into **how diet and weight loss could reset metabolic processes**, setting the stage for non-surgical approaches to reversal.

Real-World Stories: Paths to Remission

Numbers alone don't tell the whole story. The journey of **Maria Vasquez**, a retired teacher from Argentina, exemplifies the power of evidence-based lifestyle change. Diagnosed with type 2 diabetes in her late 50s, Maria struggled with fluctuating blood sugar and increasing medication. Inspired by the results of the DiRECT study and motivated by her grandchildren, she joined a local diabetes support group that emphasized whole foods, portion control, and daily walks. Within a year, Maria lost 14 kg (31 pounds), normalized her A1C, and—under her doctor's supervision—reduced her medications to almost none. Her story is echoed by thousands around the globe.

Similarly, in Japan, a country with a rising incidence of type 2 diabetes despite generally healthy diets, community programs in Okinawa have shown that **combining traditional plant-based meals with increased physical activity** can significantly improve blood sugar control, even leading to remission for many older adults. These examples highlight that, while the science is robust, **local culture and community support are also powerful agents of change**.

What Does "Reversal" Really Mean?

It's important to recognize how researchers and clinicians define reversal, or **remission**, in type 2 diabetes. The most widely accepted criteria are:

A1C (average blood sugar over 2-3 months) below 6.5%
Fasting blood glucose below 126 mg/dL
No use of diabetes medications for at least 6 months

This definition helps standardize research and clinical practice, but also points to the ongoing need for vigilance—remission is not the same as a cure, and blood sugar can rise again if healthy habits lapse.

Key Mechanisms Behind the Evidence

Why do these interventions work? Scientific studies point to several interconnected mechanisms:

- **Reduction of liver and pancreatic fat**: Excess fat in these organs disrupts insulin production and function; losing weight can restore their normal activity.
- **Improved insulin sensitivity**: Less fat and more physical activity help the body's cells respond better to insulin.
- **Metabolic flexibility**: The body regains its ability to switch between burning carbohydrates and fat, stabilizing blood sugar.

These findings are consistent across diverse populations, from the United States to India, affirming that the principles of reversal are broadly applicable—though the details may vary with culture, genetics, and environment.

```
Fact: The earlier type 2 diabetes is addressed with lifestyle changes, the
higher the chance of reversing the condition—sometimes within months.
```

The research is clear: with the right changes, many people can not only manage but potentially reverse type 2 diabetes. The stories of Maria and communities like Okinawa show that these strategies aren't confined to laboratories—they work in the real world, across cultures and continents. As we move forward, we'll dive deeper into the physiological transformations that underpin these successes, illuminating how your body can move from disease to health with the right approach.

4.3 Success Stories from Around the World

Across continents and cultures, the journey to reverse type 2 diabetes is as diverse as the people undertaking it. Yet, whether in bustling cities or rural villages, one thread unites these stories: the powerful combination of knowledge, determination, and lifestyle change. Let's explore how individuals and communities have harnessed science—and hope—to reclaim their health.

The Newcastle Miracle: Roy Taylor's Pioneering Study

In the north of England, clinical researcher **Professor Roy Taylor** and his team at Newcastle University embarked on a groundbreaking journey in the early 2010s. Their mission was bold: to see if type 2 diabetes could be reversed through radical changes in diet. The study participants, all recently diagnosed with type 2 diabetes, were placed on a very low-calorie diet—around 800 calories per day—comprised of soups and shakes for eight weeks.

The results were extraordinary. Many participants experienced significant weight loss and, more importantly, normalization of their blood sugar levels. By the study's end, a remarkable proportion no longer met the diagnostic criteria for diabetes.

Key elements of success:

- Intensive dietary intervention (very low-calorie intake)
- Close medical supervision
- Gradual reintroduction of regular foods
- Ongoing support and education

One participant, **Mark**, a 52-year-old taxi driver from Newcastle, described the transformation as "getting my future back." He recalled the sense of freedom that came when his blood sugar readings normalized, and his doctor declared he no longer needed diabetes medication. Mark's story, echoed by many others in the study, became a symbol of hope in the UK and beyond.

A South Asian Perspective: The Chennai Urban Rural Epidemiology Study

Type 2 diabetes has reached epidemic proportions in India, with genetic, dietary, and lifestyle factors contributing to the nation's high prevalence. In Chennai, Dr. **V. Mohan** and his colleagues launched the **Chennai Urban Rural Epidemiology Study (CURES)**, aiming to understand and address diabetes in the Indian context.

One of their notable initiatives was the introduction of plant-forward, culturally sensitive dietary interventions. Traditional diets—rich in whole grains, lentils, and vegetables—were promoted, while processed foods and excess sugars were minimized. The team emphasized daily physical activity, encouraging walking and yoga, deeply rooted in Indian culture.

A standout success was **Priya**, a 43-year-old schoolteacher from Chennai. Guided by local nutritionists, Priya embraced a diet centered on brown rice, dals, seasonal vegetables, and modest amounts of healthy fats. She started attending early-morning yoga classes and replaced sweetened beverages with water and buttermilk. Within six months, Priya lost 18 kilograms (about 40 pounds), her fasting glucose levels normalized, and, under her doctor's guidance, she reduced her diabetes medication. Her story was featured in local media, inspiring hundreds in her community to make similar changes.

The Tongan Community's Collective Action

Thousands of miles away on the Pacific island of **Tonga**, diabetes rates soared in recent decades due to rapid dietary shifts toward processed foods. Recognizing this crisis, local leaders and health workers implemented a culturally-tailored reversal program in partnership with international organizations.

The program encouraged the return to traditional diets—root vegetables like taro and cassava, fresh fish, and coconut—paired with community-wide physical activity initiatives such as group dance and gardening clubs. The collective nature of the effort was key; entire villages participated, supporting each other along the way.

Results:

- Widespread reduction in diabetes risk factors
- Significant weight loss and improved glucose control among participants
- Renewed pride in traditional foods and customs

The Tongan example highlights the power of community and cultural identity in tackling diabetes together—reminding us that individual change often flourishes in supportive environments.

Lessons from Around the Globe

These stories—from England, India, and Tonga—reveal patterns that transcend geography:

- **Rapid dietary changes**, when supervised and culturally adapted, can yield profound results.
- **Physical activity**, whether through yoga, walking, or traditional dance, empowers the body to process sugar more effectively.
- **Community support and cultural pride** can be as essential as any single diet or exercise plan.

More importantly, these successes show that reversal is not a remote possibility reserved for a lucky few. With the right information, tools, and support, lasting health is within reach for many.

```
FACT: In clinical studies, up to 50% of people with early-stage type 2
diabetes have achieved remission through intensive lifestyle interventions.
MEMORABLE: Type 2 diabetes reversal is possible—especially when changes are
started soon after diagnosis.
```

The science of reversal is not only written in textbooks and journal articles—it is etched in the lived experience of people worldwide. Their victories, whether personal or communal, illuminate the path forward. As we turn to the next chapter, we'll delve into the specific physiological mechanisms behind these transformations, demystifying how the body can heal itself when given the chance. The journey from disease to health continues, grounded in science and inspired by real-world triumphs.

4.4 Factors Influencing Reversibility

One of the most powerful determinants of whether type 2 diabetes can be reversed is **timing**. The earlier the intervention, the higher the chance of success. When excess blood sugar and insulin resistance are addressed swiftly, the body's metabolic machinery is less likely to suffer permanent damage. Numerous studies have shown that individuals who tackle diabetes within months or a couple of years of diagnosis—before significant pancreatic beta-cell exhaustion—are more likely to achieve remission.

For example, the groundbreaking **DiRECT (Diabetes Remission Clinical Trial)** in the UK demonstrated that people who lost substantial weight within six years of diagnosis had a remarkable chance of putting their diabetes into remission. In this study, participants followed a structured, calorie-restricted diet and received ongoing support. After just one year, nearly half of all participants achieved normal blood sugar levels without medication.

However, as the duration of type 2 diabetes increases, chronic high blood sugar can inflict lasting damage on insulin-producing cells. This underscores the need for early recognition, swift action, and ongoing vigilance.

Weight Loss and Fat Distribution

A central factor influencing reversibility is the **amount and location of excess fat**. Research shows that fat stored in the liver and pancreas—the so-called "ectopic fat"— directly impairs insulin action and production. Losing even 5-10% of body weight, especially early in the disease, can dramatically reduce this toxic fat, restoring the organs' function.

> **Visceral fat** (fat around abdominal organs) is more harmful than subcutaneous fat (fat under the skin), as it releases inflammatory signals and hormones that worsen insulin resistance.

Dramatic improvements have been observed in people who lose weight through diet, exercise, or, in some cases, bariatric surgery, reinforcing the body's capacity for recovery.

A memorable story illustrating this comes from Dr. Roy Taylor's research in Newcastle, UK. He recounts the case of Mark, a middle-aged man diagnosed with type 2 diabetes. After adopting a low-calorie diet and losing 15 kilograms, Mark's liver and pancreas fat significantly decreased, and his blood sugar normalized. Years later, he remains in remission, a testament to the transformative power of targeted weight loss.

Genetics, Ethnicity, and Cultural Background

While lifestyle change is pivotal, **genetics** and **ethnicity** also shape an individual's risk and response to intervention. Some people inherit a predisposition to insulin resistance or reduced beta-cell capacity, making reversal more challenging. Furthermore, different populations experience type 2 diabetes differently:

- **South Asians** tend to develop diabetes at lower body weights and younger ages, often with prominent visceral fat.
- **African Americans** and **Hispanic Americans** have higher rates of insulin resistance, influenced by both genetic and social determinants.
- **Indigenous populations** worldwide often face the highest rates, fueled by rapid transitions from traditional diets to Westernized, high-calorie foods.

Recognizing these differences is crucial for crafting culturally sensitive and effective reversal strategies. For example, in Japan, where white rice is a staple, recent public health campaigns have promoted brown rice and whole grains to help curb rising diabetes rates. Similarly, community-driven dietary interventions in Native American reservations have achieved promising results by reviving traditional, plant-rich foods.

Medication Use and Dependency

The **number and type of diabetes medications** a person uses can also affect reversibility. Those managing their condition with lifestyle changes alone, or on minimal medication, generally have a greater chance of remission. Over time, reliance on multiple drugs may signal more advanced disease, making reversal harder but not impossible.

Medications such as **metformin** and **GLP-1 agonists** can support remission by improving insulin sensitivity and promoting weight loss.
However, some drugs, especially those that stimulate insulin secretion, may "mask" blood sugar levels without addressing underlying resistance.

A careful, supervised reduction of medications, as lifestyle changes take effect, is a hallmark of a successful reversal process.

Commitment, Support, and Environment

Finally, the journey to reversal is shaped by **motivation, social support, and the environment**. Sustained lifestyle change is rarely achieved in isolation.

- Family involvement, peer groups, and professional coaching all increase accountability and resilience.
- Access to healthy foods, safe spaces for exercise, and culturally relevant education can tip the balance toward long-term success.

The story of "Diabetes Village" in Kerala, India, offers a compelling example. There, a community-wide initiative involving diet, exercise, and group support helped hundreds of villagers not only control but, in many cases, reverse type 2 diabetes—showcasing the transformative power of collective action.

Fact: Remission of type 2 diabetes is most likely when significant weight loss occurs soon after diagnosis—before extensive pancreatic damage takes place.

The tapestry of factors influencing diabetes reversibility is complex, weaving together biology, lifestyle, culture, and community. While not every case can be fully reversed, understanding these factors empowers individuals and families to take meaningful action. The next section will explore the practical steps—rooted in science and shaped by real-world experience—that can tip the scales toward lasting health and newfound freedom from type 2 diabetes.

4.5 Setting Realistic Expectations

Understanding the powerful promise of type 2 diabetes reversal is both inspiring and motivating. Yet, amid stories of dramatic turnarounds, it's vital to balance optimism with reality. Expectations set the stage for our journey, shaping our mindset, resilience, and willingness to persevere through inevitable ups and downs. This section explores what "reversal" truly means, the factors that influence outcomes, and why a nuanced, grounded approach is the key to lasting success.

Defining "Reversal": Beyond the Headlines

The term **reversal** often conjures images of a complete cure—no more medication, normal blood sugar, and a life free from diabetes-related worries. However, the medical community uses more precise definitions. Most experts describe reversal as achieving and maintaining **blood glucose levels below the diabetic range without the use of diabetes medications** (with the possible exception of metformin, which is sometimes continued for its cardiovascular benefits).

It's crucial to recognize that:

- **Remission** is a more accurate term than cure. The underlying susceptibility to diabetes remains, and blood sugar can rise again if healthy habits lapse.
- **Sustained lifestyle changes** are required to maintain remission; reversal is not a one-time event but an ongoing process.
- **Individual responses** vary greatly, depending on genetics, duration of diabetes, coexisting health issues, and adherence to recommended changes.

The Timeline of Change: What to Expect

Many people hope for instant results, but the body heals in its own time. Here's a general sequence of what the reversal journey may look like:

- **First Weeks:** Blood sugar levels often begin to improve quickly—sometimes within days—especially with significant dietary changes and increased activity.
- **First Few Months:** Weight loss, improved insulin sensitivity, and medication reduction may occur. Energy levels, sleep, and mood often improve.
- **6–12 Months:** Many reach a point of remission if changes are sustained, but this is not universal. Plateaus are common and require ongoing adjustments.
- **Beyond 1 Year:** Long-term maintenance becomes the focus. Occasional setbacks are normal; resilience and flexibility are essential.

It's important to communicate openly with healthcare providers throughout this timeline to adjust medications safely and monitor progress.

Success Stories: Inspiration and Reality

Maria's Story – A New Beginning in Mexico

Maria, a 54-year-old schoolteacher from Oaxaca, was diagnosed with type 2 diabetes after years of sedentary work and a diet high in refined carbohydrates. With her physician's guidance, she adopted a traditional plant-based Mexican diet rich in beans, vegetables, and whole grains, and began daily walks in her local plaza. Within six months, Maria lost 30 pounds, her blood sugar normalized, and her doctor helped her safely reduce—and eventually stop—all diabetes medications except metformin. Maria's journey shows that sustainable change is possible, especially when rooted in cultural strengths and community support.

Factors That Influence Outcomes

Despite best efforts, not everyone will experience the same degree of improvement. Several factors play a critical role:

- **Duration of diabetes:** The shorter the time since diagnosis, the higher the likelihood of remission.
- **Beta-cell function:** The pancreas's ability to produce insulin diminishes over time. Early intervention is key.
- **Degree of weight loss:** Even modest weight loss (5–10% of body weight) can have a profound impact, especially for those with central obesity.
- **Cultural and social support:** Community, family, and cultural practices can bolster success or create obstacles.

The Importance of Sustainable Change

Lasting health is built on small, consistent actions. Fad diets, extreme exercise, or drastic measures may yield quick results, but they rarely endure. Instead, focus on:

- **Personalization:** Tailor changes to your preferences, traditions, and circumstances.
- **Progress, not perfection:** Expect setbacks and use them as learning opportunities.
- **Celebrating milestones:** Every improvement—no matter how small—is a step forward.

```
- Type 2 diabetes reversal means sustained normal blood sugar without most
diabetes medications, not a permanent cure.
- Early, sustained lifestyle changes offer the greatest chance for remission.
```

Understanding what is—and isn't—possible with type 2 diabetes reversal helps set the stage for a fulfilling and realistic journey. By grounding hopes in evidence and embracing a patient, flexible attitude, you empower yourself to make meaningful changes with lasting impact. In the next section, we'll dive into the practical strategies—the daily habits, foods, and routines—that can transform hope into tangible, measurable progress.

4.6 The Path Forward

The possibility of reversing type 2 diabetes may once have sounded radical, even unattainable. For decades, the prevailing medical view was that the disease could only be "managed"—that is, kept in check with ever-increasing medications, dietary caution, and a watchful eye on complications. Yet, in recent years, this perspective has shifted dramatically. A growing body of research, combined with thousands of real-world success stories, has illuminated a new, hopeful path: type 2 diabetes, for many, can be reversed.

This evolving understanding is rooted in a deeper grasp of what drives the disease. Rather than seeing type 2 diabetes as an inevitable, progressive decline in health, scientists now recognize that its primary cause—insulin resistance—can be significantly improved. Through targeted interventions, the body's ability to regulate blood sugar can recover, sometimes to the point where blood glucose levels return to normal without the need for medication.

The Mechanisms of Reversal

To understand how reversal is possible, it helps to revisit the biology discussed earlier in this chapter. When we reduce the burden on the pancreas and the demand for insulin—primarily through dietary change and weight loss—the body's cells often become more sensitive to insulin. In some cases, the fat that accumulates around the liver and pancreas begins to recede, allowing these organs to function more effectively.

- **Caloric restriction** and **weight loss**: Landmark studies have shown that even modest weight loss (as little as 5-10% of body weight) can dramatically improve blood sugar control and, in some cases, achieve remission.
- **Low-carbohydrate and low-calorie diets**: Diets that minimize simple sugars and refined carbohydrates help reduce the need for insulin, giving the body a chance to "reset."
- **Physical activity**: Regular exercise not only burns glucose but also increases the sensitivity of muscle cells to insulin, amplifying the benefits of dietary change.

Real-World Stories: From Despair to Hope

Consider the journey of **Dr. Roy Taylor's** patients in the United Kingdom. In the landmark **DiRECT trial**, participants with recent-onset type 2 diabetes embarked on an intensive low-calorie diet under medical supervision. The results were striking: nearly half achieved remission after one year, and a significant number remained diabetes-free at two years. The study's participants described a profound sense of liberation—not just from medications, but from the mental burden of chronic illness.

In another corner of the globe, **Anita Singh**, a schoolteacher in Mumbai, found herself overwhelmed by her diagnosis and the prospect of lifelong pills. She joined a local wellness group that focused on daily walks and traditional plant-based meals low in processed sugars and oils. Within six months, her HbA1c—a measure of average blood glucose—had dropped into the normal range. Anita's story is a testament to the power of community support and culturally relevant solutions.

Historical Context: A Shift in the Paradigm

It's worth remembering how recently this possibility of reversal entered mainstream conversation. For much of the 20th century, diabetes was seen as a one-way street. It wasn't until the 21st century—with advances in metabolic research and the rise of evidence-based nutrition—that the tide began to turn.

> In 2006, the **Look AHEAD study** in the United States demonstrated that intensive lifestyle interventions could improve glycemic control and reduce medication requirements.
>
> By the late 2010s, major diabetes organizations began to acknowledge remission as a legitimate, if challenging, goal.

This shift did not occur in isolation. It was propelled by patient advocacy, cross-cultural learning, and the willingness of clinicians to challenge old dogmas. In countries as diverse as Finland, Japan, and South Africa, public health campaigns have begun to focus on early intervention and holistic care—recognizing that diabetes reversal is not just a scientific question, but a matter of social will and access.

Navigating the Road Ahead

The road to reversal is not without its challenges. It requires dedication, support, and, often, a reimagining of daily life. But as research and real-life experiences show, the rewards can be profound—not just in blood sugar numbers, but in energy, confidence, and freedom.

Key factors for success:

- Early intervention yields the best outcomes, but improvement is possible at any stage.
- Ongoing support—from healthcare providers, family, and peer groups—greatly enhances adherence and motivation.
- Individualization is critical; what works for one person may not work for another, and adjustments are part of the process.

```
Important: Remission of type 2 diabetes does not mean a "cure"—ongoing
vigilance and healthy habits are essential to maintain results.
Fact: Studies show that up to 60% of people with recent-onset type 2 diabetes
can achieve remission with intensive lifestyle changes.
```

As we have seen, the science of reversal is not just a story of medical progress, but of human resilience and hope. The path forward is illuminated by both rigorous research and the lived experience of those who have reclaimed their health. In the next chapter, we will move from theory to practice—exploring the specific foods, habits, and routines that can transform possibility into reality. With the right tools and mindset, lasting health is within reach.

5 : Food as Medicine – Building a Diabetes-Reversing Diet

5.1 Principles of a Diabetes-Reversing Diet

A diagnosis of type 2 diabetes can feel overwhelming, but the foundation of lasting health often begins at the dinner table. Scientific research and lived experience consistently show that food is a powerful form of medicine—capable not only of managing, but in many cases, reversing type 2 diabetes. In this chapter, we move beyond theory and into practice, exploring the essential principles of a diet designed to restore balance and support your body's healing potential.

Understanding the Core Principles

A diabetes-reversing diet is not a temporary fix or a rigid prescription. Instead, it draws on a deep understanding of how nutrients, meal patterns, and mindful choices can transform metabolism and blood sugar regulation. At its heart, this approach is about nourishing—not depriving—your body.

Principles of a Diabetes-Reversing Diet

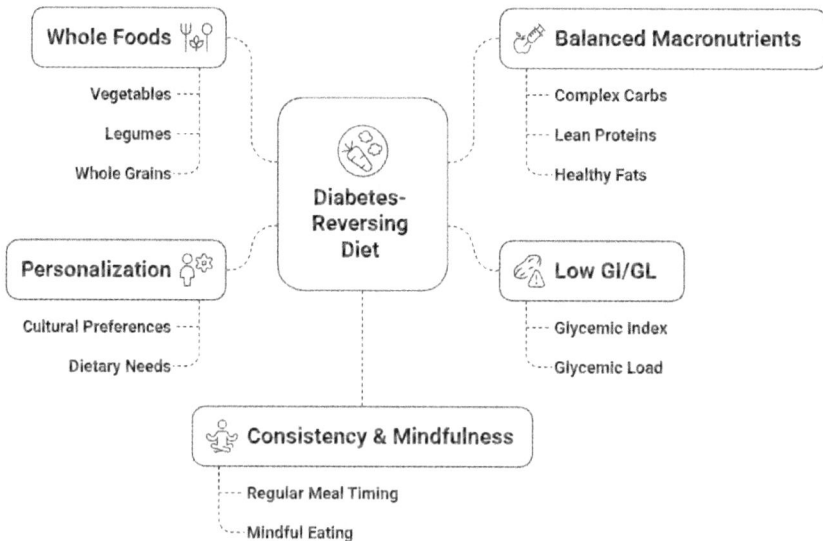

- **Focus on Whole, Minimally Processed Foods**: Foods as close as possible to their natural state—think vegetables, legumes, whole grains, nuts, and lean proteins—form the backbone of this dietary strategy. They're rich in fiber, vitamins, and minerals that support stable glucose levels.

- **Emphasize Low Glycemic Index (GI) and Glycemic Load (GL) Choices**: The glycemic index measures how quickly a food raises blood sugar, while glycemic load reflects both the quality and quantity of carbohydrate in a serving. Opting for foods with low GI and GL helps prevent blood sugar spikes.
- **Balance Macronutrients Thoughtfully**: A healthy mix of complex carbohydrates, lean proteins, and healthy fats slows digestion, smooths blood sugar fluctuations, and supports satiety.
- **Personalize for Culture and Preference**: A sustainable diabetes-reversing diet honors individual tastes, traditions, and dietary needs—whether you prefer Mediterranean, South Asian, plant-based, or other culinary heritages.
- **Prioritize Consistency and Mindfulness**: Regular meal timing and mindful eating practices help your body maintain equilibrium, reducing stress on the pancreas and improving insulin sensitivity.

A Timeline of Dietary Evolution and Diabetes

Understanding how dietary approaches to diabetes have evolved can offer perspective and inspiration:

- **Early 20th Century**: Before insulin's discovery, treatment focused on strict calorie restriction and fasting. While often effective at lowering blood sugar, these regimens were unsustainable and sometimes dangerous.
- **Mid-20th Century**: The "exchange system" emerged, allowing more flexibility with portioned food groups, but still emphasized carbohydrate control.
- **21st Century**: Advances in nutrition science highlighted the power of fiber, plant-based eating, and the importance of food quality. Culturally adapted diets and new knowledge about the glycemic index transformed diabetes management, focusing on empowerment and choice.

Real-World Stories: Food as a Turning Point

Consider the story of **Maria**, a schoolteacher from São Paulo, Brazil, diagnosed with type 2 diabetes in her late 40s. Initially, medication and vague dietary advice provided little improvement. It wasn't until Maria joined a community nutrition program—centered on unprocessed beans, fresh vegetables, and whole grains—that her numbers began to improve. By focusing on local, affordable staples and reducing sugary drinks, Maria gradually reduced her medication and regained her energy, illustrating how dietary transformation can be both practical and powerful.

Across the globe in India, **Ravi**, a long-distance runner, struggled with diabetes despite his active lifestyle. Traditional meals rich in white rice and breads kept his blood sugar high. With guidance, he switched to whole grains like millet and brown rice, added more lentils, and increased his vegetable intake. These changes, rooted in familiar foods but mindful of their glycemic impact, helped Ravi achieve stable glucose levels and rekindle his athletic ambitions.

Building Your Plate: Key Components

A diabetes-reversing meal is both visually appealing and nutritionally balanced. Here's a practical guide for constructing your plate:

Nutritional Plate Composition for Diabetes Reversal

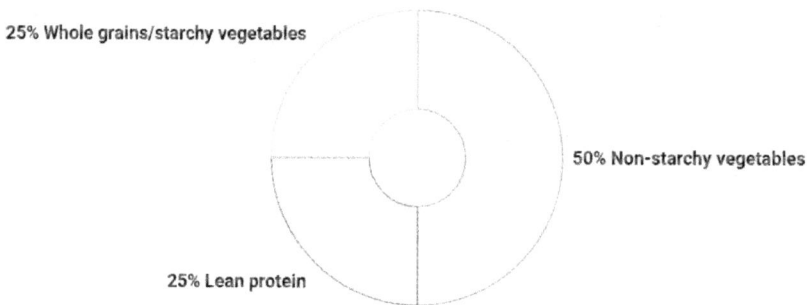

25% Whole grains/starchy vegetables

50% Non-starchy vegetables

25% Lean protein

- **Half your plate**: Non-starchy vegetables (broccoli, leafy greens, peppers)
- **One quarter**: Lean protein (fish, tofu, chicken, beans)
- **One quarter**: Whole grains or starchy vegetables (quinoa, brown rice, sweet potatoes)
- **Healthy fats**: Add a small portion of nuts, seeds, avocado, or olive oil
- **Flavor with herbs and spices**, not sugar or excessive salt

Cultural Flexibility and Global Adaptation

The path to diabetes reversal is not one-size-fits-all. In Japan, traditional diets featuring fish, seaweed, and fermented soy have been associated with lower diabetes rates, while Mediterranean patterns rich in olive oil, legumes, and fresh produce have shown significant benefits across Europe and North America. Adapting these principles to your local foods and traditions increases sustainability and enjoyment—essential ingredients for lasting change.

```
- Eating foods with a low glycemic index can reduce average blood sugar
(HbA1c) by up to 0.5-1.0%.
- Replacing just one serving of sugary drinks per day with water or
unsweetened tea can lower your diabetes risk and improve glycemic control.
```

Embracing the principles of a diabetes-reversing diet means more than following a set of rules—it's about reclaiming agency and joy in your eating habits. By combining scientific insight with cultural wisdom and personal preference, you can build a nourishing path to wellness. In the next section, we'll take a closer look at the role of specific foods and how to harness the power of the glycemic index and glycemic load to fine-tune your daily choices for optimal blood sugar control.

5.2 Understanding Carbohydrates

Carbohydrates often find themselves at the center of the conversation when it comes to type 2 diabetes. For many, they are simply "sugar" by another name, a dietary villain to be avoided at all costs. Yet, the truth is both more nuanced and empowering. Carbohydrates are not inherently harmful; in fact, they are essential for energy and cellular function. The key lies in understanding their different forms, how they interact with your body, and—most importantly—how you can make choices that support your journey toward reversing type 2 diabetes.

What Are Carbohydrates?

Carbohydrates are one of the three primary macronutrients in our diet, alongside proteins and fats. Their main role is to supply energy, as the body converts them into glucose, which fuels nearly every cell. However, not all carbohydrates are created equal. They come in a variety of forms, each with distinct effects on blood sugar:

Carbohydrate Types and Their Effects

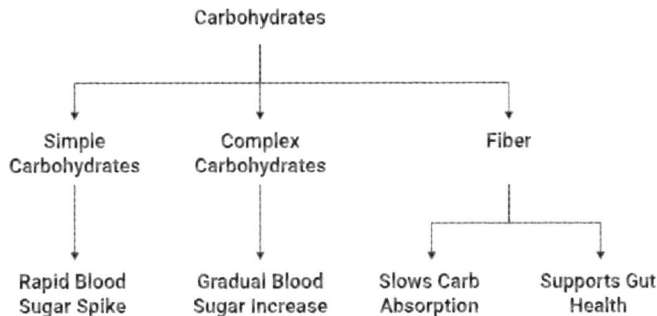

- **Simple carbohydrates**: These are quickly broken down and absorbed, causing rapid spikes in blood sugar. Examples include table sugar, honey, and most processed foods.
- **Complex carbohydrates**: Found in whole grains, legumes, vegetables, and some fruits, these are digested more slowly, leading to gradual increases in blood sugar and longer-lasting energy.
- **Fiber**: A type of carbohydrate that is indigestible. While it doesn't contribute to blood glucose, it plays a critical role in slowing absorption of other carbs and supporting gut health.

Understanding the types of carbohydrates you eat is a foundational step toward building a diabetes-reversing diet.

The Science Behind Carbohydrates and Blood Sugar

When you eat carbohydrates, your digestive system breaks them down into glucose, which enters your bloodstream. In response, your pancreas releases insulin—a hormone that helps cells absorb glucose for energy or storage. In type 2 diabetes, the body's ability to use insulin is impaired (insulin resistance), causing blood sugar levels to remain elevated.

Different carbohydrates impact blood sugar in different ways:

- **High-glycemic carbs** (like white bread or sugary drinks) cause sharp spikes in blood glucose.
- **Low-glycemic carbs** (like lentils or whole barley) release glucose more slowly, preventing sudden surges and supporting steadier energy.

This distinction is crucial; managing both the amount and the type of carbohydrates is a proven approach to improving blood sugar control and, over time, reducing medication dependency.

A Personal Story: Maria's Turning Point

Consider Maria, a 54-year-old teacher from the Philippines. For years, Maria believed that rice—a staple in her culture—was an unavoidable part of every meal. After being diagnosed with type 2 diabetes, she felt overwhelmed by conflicting advice. It was only when she learned about complex carbohydrates that she began replacing white rice with brown rice and adding more legumes and leafy greens to her meals. Within months, her blood sugar stabilized, her energy improved, and her doctor was able to reduce her medication. Maria's story is a testament to the transformative power of understanding—not eliminating—carbohydrates.

Historical Perspective: Carbohydrates Through the Ages

The relationship between humans and carbohydrates is centuries old. Ancient civilizations, from the maize growers of Mesoamerica to the millet farmers of Africa, relied on complex carbohydrates as dietary staples. These foods were typically unrefined and high in fiber, contributing to lower rates of chronic disease. It was only with the advent of industrial food processing in the 20th century that refined sugars and flours became widespread, paralleling the global rise in type 2 diabetes.

This historical shift underscores an important point: it is not carbohydrates themselves, but the *type* and *processing* of those carbohydrates that matters. Reclaiming traditional, whole-food sources of carbohydrates can be a powerful strategy for restoring health.

Carbohydrates in a Global Context

Across the world, different cultures have developed healthy relationships with carbohydrates:

> In **India**, traditional diets feature whole grains like millet and quinoa, alongside pulses and vegetables, supporting balanced blood sugar.
>
> In **Japan**, meals center on small portions of rice paired with vegetables, fish, and fermented foods, resulting in lower rates of metabolic disease.

These examples highlight that a diabetes-reversing diet does not mean giving up cultural foods—it means making mindful swaps and embracing traditional wisdom.

Practical Tips for Choosing Carbohydrates

To make carbohydrates work for you, consider these strategies:

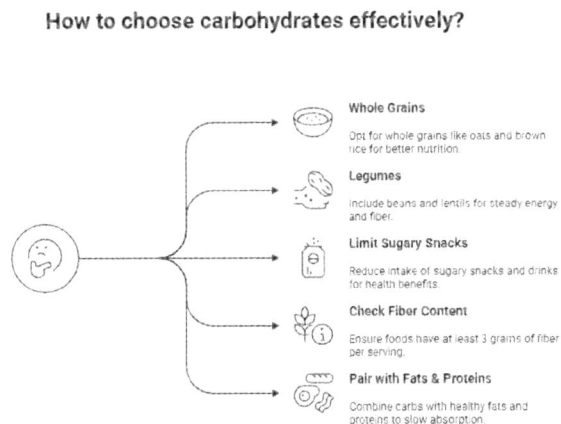

How to choose carbohydrates effectively?

Whole Grains
Opt for whole grains like oats and brown rice for better nutrition.

Legumes
Include beans and lentils for steady energy and fiber.

Limit Sugary Snacks
Reduce intake of sugary snacks and drinks for health benefits.

Check Fiber Content
Ensure foods have at least 3 grams of fiber per serving.

Pair with Fats & Proteins
Combine carbs with healthy fats and proteins to slow absorption.

- Choose **whole grains** (such as oats, barley, and brown rice) over refined grains.
- Incorporate **beans, lentils, and legumes** for steady energy and extra fiber.
- Limit **sugary snacks** and sweetened beverages.
- Read labels for **fiber content**—aim for foods with at least 3 grams per serving.
- Pair carbohydrates with **healthy fats** and **proteins** to slow absorption.

The Takeaway

Carbohydrates are neither friend nor foe—they are a tool, and your understanding of them is the key. By choosing complex, minimally processed carbs and balancing them with fiber, protein, and healthy fats, you lay the foundation for lasting health and diabetes reversal.

```
Fact: Fiber-rich carbohydrates not only slow blood sugar spikes but also
support gut health, reduce inflammation, and promote satiety, making them
essential in a diabetes-reversing diet.
```

As we move forward, we'll explore how to use the glycemic index and glycemic load to further refine your carbohydrate choices—empowering you to personalize your diet for optimal blood sugar control and greater vitality.

5.3 Protein and Healthy Fats

When the conversation around diabetes and nutrition begins, carbohydrates tend to dominate the spotlight. Yet, **protein**—long revered as the building block of life—plays an equally vital, if quieter, role in the path to reversing type 2 diabetes. Unlike carbohydrates, protein has a minimal direct impact on blood sugar. Instead, it helps stabilize glucose levels by slowing the absorption of sugars from other foods and promoting satiety, making it less likely that you'll overindulge in high-glycemic fare.

Consider the story of **Carlos**, a 52-year-old teacher from San Antonio, Texas. Diagnosed with type 2 diabetes in his forties, Carlos felt overwhelmed by dietary restrictions. After consulting a nutritionist, he began replacing his typical high-carb breakfasts with scrambled eggs and sautéed spinach. Within weeks, Carlos noticed not only more stable blood sugar readings but also greater energy and fewer cravings throughout the day.

The Science Behind Protein's Power

Protein's influence extends beyond mere blood sugar control. When consumed, protein triggers the release of hormones like **GLP-1** and **PYY**, which promote fullness and help regulate appetite. This can be especially helpful for those seeking weight loss—

a key factor in reversing insulin resistance. Moreover, adequate protein intake protects lean muscle mass, which often declines with age or rapid weight loss, and is crucial for maintaining metabolic health.

Best Protein Sources for Diabetes Management

- **Lean meats**: Skinless poultry, turkey, and lean cuts of beef or pork
- **Fish and seafood**: Salmon, sardines, mackerel, and shrimp (rich in omega-3s)
- **Eggs**: Versatile and nutrient-dense, eggs are a powerhouse for satiety
- **Low-fat dairy**: Greek yogurt, cottage cheese, and kefir
- **Plant-based proteins**: Beans, lentils, tofu, tempeh, and edamame

For those following plant-based diets, the next section will offer a deep dive into maximizing protein from non-animal sources.

Healthy Fats: The Right Kind of Energy

If protein is the unsung hero, **healthy fats** are often the misunderstood ally in the diabetes-reversing toolkit. For decades, dietary fat was wrongly blamed for a host of health woes. Today, science has clearly distinguished between harmful trans and saturated fats and the beneficial unsaturated fats that support heart and metabolic health.

Healthy fats—especially monounsaturated and polyunsaturated varieties—play a critical role in managing type 2 diabetes. They slow gastric emptying, further moderating blood sugar spikes, and provide long-lasting energy. These fats are also essential for absorbing fat-soluble vitamins (A, D, E, and K) and supporting anti-inflammatory processes throughout the body.

Top Sources of Healthy Fats

- **Avocados:** Rich in monounsaturated fats, fiber, and antioxidants
- **Nuts and seeds:** Almonds, walnuts, chia, flax, and pumpkin seeds supply omega-3s and protein
- **Olive oil:** A Mediterranean staple, loaded with heart-healthy monounsaturated fats
- **Fatty fish:** Salmon, trout, and sardines offer a potent dose of omega-3 fatty acids
- **Nut butters:** Peanut and almond butter (in moderation, and with no added sugar or hydrogenated oils)

A Global Perspective: The Mediterranean Model

Across the globe, communities in the Mediterranean region have long enjoyed some of the world's lowest rates of chronic disease, including type 2 diabetes. Their secret? A diet abundant in olive oil, nuts, fish, legumes, and fresh vegetables. The **PREDIMED Study**—a landmark trial conducted in Spain—demonstrated that participants following a Mediterranean diet with extra virgin olive oil or nuts experienced a significant reduction in the risk of developing type 2 diabetes compared to those on a low-fat diet.

This historical example underscores how dietary fats, when chosen wisely, can be powerful medicine rather than a foe.

Balancing Protein and Healthy Fats: Practical Strategies

Making protein and healthy fats the cornerstone of your meals doesn't require a complete overhaul of your kitchen. Instead, small, consistent changes can yield profound results:

- **Start your day with protein:** Swap refined cereals for eggs, Greek yogurt, or a lentil-based breakfast.
- **Add healthy fats:** Top salads with avocado or a handful of nuts; drizzle roasted vegetables with olive oil.
- **Snack smart:** Replace chips and crackers with a boiled egg or a small portion of unsalted nuts.
- **Prioritize fish:** Aim for at least two servings of fatty fish per week for omega-3 benefits.
- **Watch portion sizes:** Even healthy fats are calorie-dense, so use moderation to avoid weight gain.

Key Takeaways

```
- Protein and healthy fats stabilize blood sugar and promote fullness,
reducing the likelihood of overeating.
- Choosing the right kinds of fats—especially unsaturated fats—can improve
heart and metabolic health in people with type 2 diabetes.
```

Protein and healthy fats are essential pillars in the fight against type 2 diabetes, offering both metabolic and practical benefits. By focusing on these nutrient-rich foods and drawing inspiration from diverse global traditions, anyone can create a sustainable, diabetes-reversing plan. Next, we'll shift our attention to vegetarian and plant-based strategies, ensuring that everyone—regardless of dietary preference—has the tools to thrive on the path to lasting health.

5.4 Cultural Approaches to Healthy Eating

Across continents and centuries, cultures have crafted unique solutions for nourishing the body—a testament to human ingenuity and adaptability. As we explore how food acts as medicine in the journey to reverse type 2 diabetes, it's essential to honor and learn from these diverse traditions. By embracing cultural approaches, we not only make dietary changes more enjoyable but also more sustainable, respectful, and effective.

The Mediterranean Model: A Blueprint for Longevity

The **Mediterranean diet** has become a gold standard in diabetes prevention and reversal for good reason. Rooted in the eating habits of countries like Greece, Italy, and Spain, this approach emphasizes:

- Abundant fruits and vegetables
- Whole grains, legumes, and nuts
- Olive oil as the primary fat source
- Moderate consumption of fish and poultry
- Limited intake of red meats and sweets

What makes the Mediterranean diet so powerful is its balance: meals are rich in fiber, healthy fats, and phytonutrients, all of which help stabilize blood sugar. In the famous **Seven Countries Study** led by Ancel Keys in the 1950s, populations around the Mediterranean exhibited remarkably low rates of heart disease and diabetes despite consuming moderate amounts of fat. Their secret lay in the types of fats they chose, their reliance on plant-based foods, and the rhythm of shared, unhurried meals.

Maria's Story:

Maria, a 62-year-old from southern Italy, faced rising blood sugar after years of urban living and processed foods. Returning to her roots, she began cooking traditional dishes—like chickpea stew, grilled vegetables, and fresh tomato salads—replacing white bread with whole-grain loaves and using olive oil instead of butter. Over several months, her glucose levels normalized, and her energy soared. Maria's experience illustrates how cultural food wisdom can help reclaim health.

Asian Traditions: Harmony, Variety, and Balance

Many Asian culinary traditions center on **balance**—not just in flavors, but in nutrition. In Japan, the traditional **washoku** approach highlights:

- Plenty of vegetables, seaweed, and soy-based proteins
- Modest portions of rice or other grains

- Fish as a regular protein source
- Minimal use of added sugars or oils

The Japanese concept of **hara hachi bu**—"eat until you are 80% full"—encourages mindful eating and portion control, both critical for blood sugar management. Similarly, in India, centuries-old Ayurvedic dietary principles emphasize whole grains like millet and barley, a rainbow of vegetables, and legumes, often accompanied by beneficial spices such as turmeric and fenugreek, which have been shown to aid glucose metabolism.

Latin American Flavors: Harnessing Indigenous Superfoods

In many Latin American cultures, traditional diets are built around **whole, unrefined foods** such as beans, corn, squash, and a variety of fresh produce. Staples like **quinoa, amaranth, and black beans** supply slow-digesting carbohydrates and ample fiber, helping to blunt blood sugar spikes. Salsas, guacamole, and roasted vegetables add flavor without relying on processed sugars or unhealthy fats.

The indigenous peoples of the Andes, for example, have cultivated quinoa for thousands of years—a seed with a low glycemic index and complete protein profile. When these time-honored foods are prioritized over modern ultra-processed fare, blood sugar control improves dramatically.

Adapting Traditions for Modern Health

Cultural heritage is a powerful ally in diabetes reversal, but adaptation is sometimes necessary:

- Swap white rice for brown, wild rice, or ancient grains.
- Use traditional spices and herbs to enhance flavor, reducing the need for added salt or sugar.
- Choose grilling, steaming, or roasting over deep-frying.
- Practice communal meals, savoring food and fostering social connection, which can reduce stress and support better choices.

Building a Personal, Culturally-Rooted Plan

No single diet fits everyone. The most effective diabetes-reversing plan is one that feels familiar, joyful, and meaningful. Integrating family recipes, honoring food rituals, and making gradual improvements can transform daunting changes into a source of pride and connection.

- Start by identifying 2-3 traditional dishes you love.

- Modify ingredients for better glycemic control (e.g., use whole grains, increase vegetables).
- Involve family or community members in meal preparation.
- Celebrate progress, not perfection.

```
- Traditional diets—rich in whole foods and low in refined sugars—consistently
correlate with lower rates of type 2 diabetes worldwide.
- Culturally familiar meals, when adapted for health, are more likely to lead
to lasting lifestyle change.
```

By drawing inspiration from diverse cultural traditions, we can create a diabetes-reversing diet that is both nourishing and sustainable. These approaches remind us that food is not just fuel, but a profound expression of identity and community. In the following section, we'll delve deeper into plant-based strategies, ensuring those on vegetarian or vegan paths have robust, evidence-based tools for optimal blood sugar control.

5.5 Meal Planning and Preparation

Successful reversal of type 2 diabetes hinges on more than isolated food choices—it's about orchestrating entire days and weeks of balanced, nourishing meals. **Meal planning** becomes a cornerstone, allowing you to anticipate needs, avoid impulsive eating, and ensure every bite serves your body's healing journey. The goal is not deprivation, but empowerment; you're designing a life where food becomes an ally rather than an adversary.

- **Consistency matters:** Eating at regular intervals helps maintain stable blood sugar.
- **Portion control:** Thoughtful serving sizes prevent overconsumption and wild glucose swings.
- **Variety:** Rotating proteins, vegetables, and grains ensures broad nutrient coverage and keeps meals exciting.

Consider the story of **Carlos**, a 52-year-old teacher from Mexico City. After his diagnosis, he struggled with erratic meals—sometimes skipping breakfast, other days indulging in late-night snacks. Guided by a diabetes educator, he began prepping weekly menus, batch-cooking beans and chopping vegetables ahead of time. Within weeks, his energy surged, and his glucose readings began to stabilize. Carlos's journey underscores a universal truth: planning isn't just about food; it's about reclaiming agency over your health.

Setting Up for Success: Kitchen and Pantry Essentials

Before diving into recipes or menus, setting up your environment is crucial. A well-stocked kitchen makes healthy choices effortless and minimizes reliance on processed foods.

- **Whole grains:** Quinoa, brown rice, barley, and steel-cut oats offer fiber and slow-release energy.
- **Lean proteins:** Skinless poultry, fish, tofu, and legumes are excellent staples.
- **Colorful produce:** Aim for a rainbow—leafy greens, berries, cruciferous vegetables, and root crops.
- **Healthy fats:** Olive oil, avocado, nuts, and seeds provide satiety and heart health benefits.
- **Herbs and spices:** Enhance flavor without excess salt or sugar.

Across cultures, food traditions have long championed such staples. In the Mediterranean region, for instance, families gather around tables brimming with legumes, vegetables, and olive oil—an approach now recognized globally for its diabetes-fighting potential.

Crafting a Diabetes-Reversing Meal Plan

A thoughtfully designed meal plan balances **glycemic index (GI)** and **glycemic load (GL)**, carbohydrates, proteins, and healthy fats. Here's how to begin:

- **Assess your baseline.** Review recent meals and snacks. Identify high-GI foods and processed items that need replacing.
- **Map out your week.** Choose 2–3 breakfast, lunch, and dinner options to rotate, mixing in seasonal produce and local flavors.
- **Batch cook and prep.** Prepare grains, beans, and roasted vegetables in bulk. Portion out ingredients for grab-and-go meals.
- **Build balanced plates.** Fill half your plate with non-starchy vegetables, a quarter with lean protein, and a quarter with whole grains or legumes.
- **Plan snacks purposefully.** Stock up on nuts, seeds, plain yogurt, and fresh fruit for steady energy between meals.

Meal Preparation: Practical Tips for Everyday Life

- **Use visual cues:** Store pre-cut vegetables at eye level in the fridge for easy access.
- **Embrace slow cookers or instant pots:** These tools save time and allow for healthy, one-pot meals.

- **Label portions:** Use containers to manage serving sizes and reduce guesswork.
- **Schedule meal prep:** Block off a weekly time, making it a non-negotiable self-care ritual.

For those with busy schedules, small adjustments—like preparing overnight oats or assembling salad jars—can make a world of difference. The key is consistency over perfection.

Navigating Social Events and Eating Out

Social gatherings and restaurant meals need not derail your progress. Preparation and mindfulness are your best allies:

- **Preview menus:** Many restaurants post nutritional information online.
- **Communicate needs:** Don't hesitate to request modifications—sauces on the side, extra veggies, or whole grain substitutions.
- **Prioritize protein and fiber:** These help blunt glucose spikes, even in unfamiliar settings.

A Timeless Reminder

Historical records from ancient China and Greece reveal the wisdom of communal meal preparation—families and villages would gather to cook, share, and support each other's health. This collective approach fostered accountability and resilience, values that remain relevant as you build your own diabetes-reversing routine.

`Remember: Consistent meal timing and preparation are proven to help maintain blood sugar stability and reduce the risk of diabetes complications.`

Strategic meal planning and preparation transform healthy eating from a daunting task into a sustainable lifestyle. By taking charge of your kitchen and routine, you lay the groundwork for lasting blood sugar control and overall well-being. In the next section, we'll dive deeper into tailored plant-based approaches, equipping vegetarians and vegans with practical strategies for thriving on their diabetes-reversing journey.

6 : The Glycemic Index & Load – Mastering Blood Sugar Control

6.1 What Are the Glycemic Index and Load?

Imagine two friends, Maria and David, both diagnosed with type 2 diabetes. One morning, Maria enjoys a bowl of quick-cooking oats, while David opts for a sugary breakfast cereal. An hour later, Maria feels steady and focused, while David is irritable and sluggish. The difference? Their breakfasts had dramatically different effects on their blood sugar—an effect governed by the **glycemic index**.

The **glycemic index (GI)** is a ranking system developed in the early 1980s by Dr. David Jenkins and his team at the University of Toronto. The GI measures how quickly carbohydrates in foods raise blood glucose levels after eating, compared to pure glucose (which is given a GI of 100). Foods are classified as:

Glycemic Index Food Hierarchy

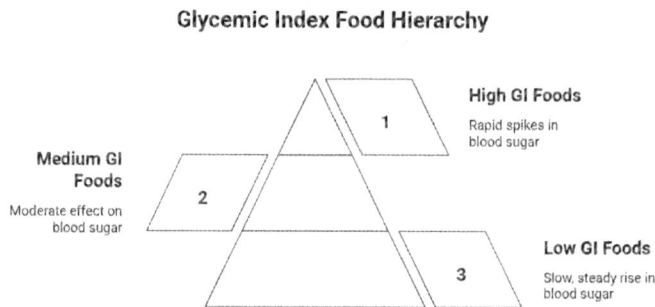

- **Low GI (55 or less):** Includes foods like lentils, most fruits, and whole grains. These cause a slow, steady rise in blood sugar.
- **Medium GI (56–69):** Examples include sweet corn, bananas, and some brown rices.
- **High GI (70 or more):** Such as white bread, instant rice, and many processed cereals, which cause rapid spikes in blood sugar.

By choosing foods with a lower GI, individuals can better manage their blood sugar levels, reducing the risk of spikes and crashes—a crucial step in reversing type 2 diabetes.

Glycemic Load: The Bigger Picture

While GI tells us how fast a carbohydrate turns into sugar, it doesn't consider the **amount** of carbohydrate in a typical serving. Enter the **glycemic load (GL)**—a more practical measure for real-life eating.

Glycemic load combines both the quality (GI) and quantity of carbohydrates in a serving of food:

GL = (GI x grams of carbohydrate per serving) ÷ 100

This means that even a food with a high GI may not always have a huge impact on blood sugar if you eat only a small portion. For example, watermelon has a high GI but a low GL because it contains little carbohydrate per serving.

GL categories:

- **Low GL (10 or less)**
- **Medium GL (11–19)**
- **High GL (20 or more)**

This dual approach allows for more nuanced, sustainable choices. For example, carrots have a relatively high GI, but because a typical serving has few carbohydrates, their GL is low. This nuance is liberating for anyone managing diabetes: it's not only what you eat, but how much.

Why Glycemic Index and Load Matter for Lasting Health

For those seeking to reverse type 2 diabetes, mastering GI and GL is a game-changer. Research across cultures—from Mediterranean countries with their emphasis on beans and whole grains to East Asian diets rich in sweet potatoes and brown rice—shows that populations with a diet focused on low-GI, low-GL foods have lower rates of type 2 diabetes and fewer complications.

A study in Australia found that Aboriginal communities who returned to traditional diets of bush foods (naturally low GI) experienced dramatic improvements in blood sugar, cholesterol, and even body weight within weeks. This historical anecdote underscores the power of aligning modern science with traditional wisdom.

Making It Work for You

To harness the power of GI and GL, consider these practical strategies:

- **Swap high-GI foods for low-GI alternatives:** Choose oats over cornflakes, sweet potatoes over white potatoes, and whole fruits over fruit juices.
- **Be mindful of portion size:** Even healthy foods can raise blood sugar if eaten in excess.
- **Combine foods wisely:** Pair carbohydrates with protein, healthy fats, or fiber to slow absorption and lower the overall GI and GL of a meal.

- **Plan ahead:** Use online databases or smartphone apps to check the GI and GL of your favorite foods.

```
Fact: Low-GI diets can reduce HbA1c by 0.5-1%, offering glycemic control
comparable to some diabetes medications.
Important: Glycemic load is often a better predictor of blood sugar response
than glycemic index alone.
```

In summary, understanding and applying the concepts of **glycemic index** and **glycemic load** provides a powerful framework for making everyday food choices that support blood sugar control and long-term health. By focusing on both the type and amount of carbohydrate, you can tailor your diet to reverse type 2 diabetes safely and sustainably.

As we move forward, we'll explore how to turn this knowledge into practical meal planning—ensuring that every bite you take supports your journey to lasting wellness.

6.2 How Foods Rank: High, Medium, Low

Demystifying Food Rankings: What High, Medium, and Low Really Mean

Now that you're familiar with the twin pillars of **glycemic index (GI)** and **glycemic load (GL)**, it's time to bring these concepts to life. Learning how foods are classified as high, medium, or low on the glycemic scale is the key to transforming your daily choices—from the bread you toast in the morning to the snacks you reach for in the afternoon—into powerful tools for blood sugar control.

Understanding the Numbers

Foods are assigned a **glycemic index** value on a scale from 0 to 100. These values reflect how rapidly a food causes your blood sugar to rise compared to pure glucose, which is given a GI of 100. The rankings are generally grouped as follows:

Low GI: 55 or less
Medium GI: 56–69
High GI: 70 or above

But just as important is the **glycemic load**, which factors in not only the quality but the quantity of carbohydrate in a typical serving. Here's how GL is ranked:

Low GL: 10 or less
Medium GL: 11–19
High GL: 20 or more

By understanding both systems, you gain a fuller picture. For example, watermelon has a high GI but a low GL because you'd have to eat a lot of it to get a significant carbohydrate load.

The Story of the White Bagel and the Lentil Soup

Let's bring these numbers to life with a real-world example. Meet Anita, a 52-year-old schoolteacher recently diagnosed with type 2 diabetes. Like many, her go-to breakfast was a toasted white bagel with cream cheese—a quick, satisfying start to her busy mornings. But after learning about GI, she discovered that her beloved bagel had a GI above 70 and a high GL, meaning it spiked her blood sugar fast and hard.

On the advice of her diabetes educator, Anita started swapping her bagel for a bowl of lentil soup (GI around 30, low GL). Within weeks, she noticed her midmorning energy crashes faded. Her blood sugar readings stabilized. This simple food swap—guided by GI and GL—helped her regain control over her mornings and, by extension, her health.

High GI/GL Foods: The Fast Track to Spikes

Foods high on the GI/GL scale are digested and absorbed rapidly, causing swift, pronounced spikes in blood sugar. These include:

- White bread and bagels
- Most breakfast cereals (e.g., cornflakes, puffed rice)
- Baked potatoes, French fries
- White rice and many processed rice products
- Sweets, candies, and sugary drinks

Across the globe, the increased popularity of Western-style fast foods—often high GI/GL—has paralleled rising type 2 diabetes rates, especially in countries like India and China where traditional diets once emphasized whole grains and legumes with lower GI.

Medium GI/GL Foods: Proceed with Caution

Medium GI/GL foods raise blood sugar more moderately. While not off-limits, they require portion mindfulness:

- Basmati rice
- Sweet corn
- Pineapple
- Rye and pita bread

In Mediterranean countries, where meals often pair medium GI grains with heart-healthy fats and vegetables, type 2 diabetes rates remain lower, highlighting the power of food synergy.

Low GI/GL Foods: Your Allies in Control

Low GI/GL foods are digested and absorbed slowly, providing sustained energy and minimizing blood sugar fluctuations. These are the foundation for reversing type 2 diabetes:

- Most non-starchy vegetables (broccoli, spinach, tomatoes)
- Legumes (lentils, chickpeas, black beans)
- Whole, minimally processed grains (steel-cut oats, barley)
- Nuts and seeds
- Dairy, especially unsweetened yogurt

Consider the case of the Okinawan diet in Japan, rich in sweet potatoes (GI 44) and legumes. For decades, this population has enjoyed some of the world's lowest rates of diabetes and the longest lifespans, a testament to the power of low GI/GL eating patterns.

How to Make Smart Swaps

Shifting to lower GI/GL foods doesn't mean sacrificing flavor or satisfaction. Here are simple swaps to get you started:

- Replace white rice with quinoa or barley.
- Trade white bread for whole grain or sprouted bread.
- Enjoy fruit with a handful of nuts to lower the overall GI of your snack.
- Choose steel-cut oats instead of instant oatmeal.

Key Takeaways

- **High GI/GL foods** spike blood sugar quickly and should be minimized.
- **Medium GI/GL foods** can fit into a balanced diet with careful portion control.
- **Low GI/GL foods** are the foundation for stable blood sugar and lasting health.

Combining foods—such as pairing carbs with protein, fat, or fiber—can lower the overall glycemic impact of a meal.

Fact: Consistently choosing low or medium GI/GL foods can reduce A1C levels—an average blood sugar marker—by up to 0.5%, a clinically significant change for many living with type 2 diabetes.

As you reflect on these rankings, remember: knowledge is only powerful when put into action. By choosing foods that work with, not against, your body's natural rhythms, you are actively rewriting your health story—one meal at a time.

In the next section, we'll turn this knowledge into practical meal planning. You'll discover how to craft breakfasts, lunches, and dinners that keep your blood sugar steady, your energy high, and your path toward reversing type 2 diabetes clear and achievable.

6.3 Strategies for Lowering GI/GL in Meals

When it comes to lowering the **glycemic index (GI)** and **glycemic load (GL)** of your meals, small changes can yield profound results. These changes are not about deprivation but about empowerment—giving you practical tools to redesign your plate for improved blood sugar control and, ultimately, a reversal of type 2 diabetes.

Combining Macronutrients for Steady Energy

Carbohydrates have the most significant impact on blood sugar, but what you eat with them matters just as much. Pairing carbs with **protein** and **healthy fats** slows down digestion, leading to a gentler rise in blood glucose.

- Add a handful of nuts or seeds to oatmeal or yogurt.
- Include lean proteins like eggs, tofu, or grilled chicken with rice or pasta dishes.
- Choose avocado or olive oil-based dressings over sugary sauces.

Choosing Whole Over Refined

Whole grains, legumes, and minimally processed foods have a lower GI compared to their refined counterparts. The fiber, intact plant structure, and natural nutrients all contribute to a slower, more controlled release of glucose.

- Swap white rice for brown rice, quinoa, or barley.
- Select whole fruit over fruit juice or sweetened fruit products.
- Replace white bread with 100% whole grain or sprouted grain bread.

Cooking Methods Matter

How you cook your food can change its GI. For example, overcooking pasta or rice causes starches to break down more, raising their GI.

- Cook pasta al dente rather than soft and mushy.
- Steam or roast vegetables instead of boiling them until soft.
- Allow potatoes to cool after cooking—the cooling process increases **resistant starch**, which lowers GI.

Smart Food Pairings: The Art of Balance

Mixing low-GI foods with higher-GI options can lower the overall glycemic impact of a meal. It is not about eliminating all high-GI items, but balancing your plate.

- Add a generous portion of leafy greens to meals with potatoes or bread.
- Pair tropical fruits (like pineapple) with cottage cheese or Greek yogurt.
- Combine beans or lentils with rice to create a lower GI meal than rice alone.

Portion Control: The Unsung Hero

What you eat is important, but how much you eat is equally critical. Even low-GI foods can lead to a spike if eaten in excess. Measuring portions and using smaller plates can help you keep GL in check.

- Serve grains and starchy vegetables as a side, not the main feature.
- Fill half your plate with non-starchy vegetables.
- Use the "plate method": 1/2 vegetables, 1/4 lean protein, 1/4 whole grains.

Global Perspective: South Asian Approaches

In India, white rice is a staple, but families often combine it with fiber-rich lentils (dal), vegetables, and yogurt. This meal structure—known as a **thali**—demonstrates how strategic food pairings can mitigate the high GI of certain staples and create a more balanced, diabetes-friendly meal.

Snack Smarter

Snacking needn't be a blood sugar minefield. Opt for options that combine fiber, fat, and protein:

- Raw vegetables with hummus.
- Apple slices with almond butter.
- A small bowl of mixed nuts.

Beverages: The Hidden Culprit

Remember, drinks can be stealthy sources of sugar and high GI. Water, unsweetened herbal teas, and sparkling water are best for blood sugar stability.

Key Takeaways for Everyday Success

- Mix carbs with protein and fat for gentler blood sugar rises.
- Prioritize whole, minimally processed foods.
- Control portions and balance your plate.

- • Choose cooking methods that preserve structure and fiber.
- • Pair foods creatively to reduce the glycemic impact.

```
- Pasta cooked al dente has a lower GI (around 50) than overcooked pasta (up
to 70).
- Combining fiber-rich foods with carbohydrates can lower the overall glycemic
load of a meal.
```

As you put these strategies into practice, remember that the goal is to find a sustainable, enjoyable way of eating that works for your lifestyle and cultural preferences. By mastering the art of lowering GI and GL in your meals, you're not just managing your diabetes—you're reclaiming the pleasure of eating and taking a powerful step toward lasting health.

In our next section, we'll explore tailored plant-based nutrition strategies, providing practical approaches for vegetarians and anyone seeking to harness the power of plants in reversing type 2 diabetes. This journey is about more than numbers; it's about nourishing your body and spirit in every bite.

6.4 Global Perspectives on GI/GL

Imagine stepping into a bustling open-air market in Mumbai, where the scent of fresh turmeric and coriander mingles with tropical fruits, or walking through a Parisian bakery, the shelves lined with golden baguettes and flaky pastries. While food is inseparable from culture, how different societies understand and manage the **glycemic index (GI)** and **glycemic load (GL)** can profoundly shape their approach to type 2 diabetes. As we deepen our understanding of these tools, it's essential to recognize that the journey to blood sugar control—like the foods we eat—is not one-size-fits-all.

Why GI and GL Matter Worldwide

The concepts of GI and GL have traveled far from their origins in Canadian laboratories in the early 1980s. Today, they underpin dietary guidelines from Australia to Japan, influencing everything from hospital menus to street food. Yet, how people apply them varies based on local ingredients, culinary traditions, and even economic realities.

Glycemic Index (GI) measures how quickly a food raises blood sugar.
Glycemic Load (GL) considers both the GI and the amount of carbohydrate in a serving, offering a more practical picture.

Both are critical, but context matters. For some, rice is a daily staple; for others, bread or maize forms the foundation of meals. Understanding GI and GL through a global lens helps us adapt their principles to our own heritage and habits.

The Australian Experience: Pioneer of Low-GI Living

Australia was among the earliest adopters of low-GI principles for diabetes management. In the 1990s, nutritionist **Professor Jennie Brand-Miller** and her team at the University of Sydney popularized the concept, developing one of the world's largest databases of GI-tested foods. Australian supermarkets now label many products as "low GI," and dietitians routinely incorporate GI/GL advice into care plans.

Japan: Tradition Meets Science

Japan's approach to diabetes and GI/GL offers a striking example of cultural adaptation. The Japanese diet, rich in rice and noodles, initially presented a challenge. However, Japanese researchers and chefs began to explore ways to lower the GI of traditional meals without sacrificing taste or heritage.

Use of mixed grains (e.g., barley with rice) to reduce overall GI.

Inclusion of fiber-rich seaweeds and vegetables.

Emphasis on portion control—a longstanding cultural practice—naturally helps mitigate GL.

The result? Japan has some of the world's lowest rates of obesity and, until recent decades, type 2 diabetes. As Westernized diets have crept in, so too have higher-GI foods and rising diabetes rates, underscoring the importance of both tradition and innovation.

Latin America: Maize, Beans, and Blood Sugar

Across Latin America, corn (maize) is a dietary staple, especially in the form of tortillas. While maize itself has a moderate GI, traditional meals nearly always pair it with beans—a powerful, low-GI food packed with fiber and protein.

A Universal Principle: Adaptation Over Perfection

What unites these global stories is not the strict avoidance of any one food, but the creative adaptation of GI/GL principles to local traditions. Whether it's swapping out sticky white rice for barley in Tokyo, enjoying dhal with whole grain chapati in Mumbai, or pairing corn with legumes in Mexico City, the key is:

Awareness: Understanding how foods affect blood sugar.

Balance: Combining high- and low-GI foods for a healthy GL.

Cultural Respect: Preserving heritage while embracing evidence-based change.

Key Global Takeaways

Many traditional diets naturally incorporate low-GI, high-fiber foods.

Combining carbohydrates with proteins, fats, or fiber-rich ingredients lowers the overall glycemic impact of a meal.

Small changes—such as choosing whole grains or adjusting portion sizes—can have a profound effect on blood sugar control.

```
Swapping just one high-GI staple (like white rice) for a lower-GI alternative
(like lentils or barley) can significantly improve blood sugar control and
reduce long-term diabetes risk.
```

```
Pairing carbohydrates with protein, fiber, or healthy fats slows digestion and
helps keep blood sugar steady—a principle recognized in traditional cuisines
worldwide.
```

Exploring global perspectives on GI and GL reveals that lasting health is best achieved through adaptation, not deprivation. By honoring our cultural roots and blending them with science, we make diabetes management both meaningful and sustainable. As we move forward, let's put this global wisdom into daily practice, transforming knowledge into the foundation for real, lasting change.

In the next section, we'll translate these insights into actionable steps—building your personal GI/GL toolkit to master blood sugar control, meal by meal.

6.5 Reading Labels and Making Choices

As you step into the grocery store, the landscape transforms into a patchwork of options—some promising health, others masking hidden sugar spikes. Understanding the **glycemic index (GI)** and **glycemic load (GL)** is just the beginning; the true art lies in applying this knowledge every time you make a food choice. Reading food labels and making conscious selections become powerful tools in your journey towards reversing type 2 diabetes.

Decoding the Nutrition Label: Your First Line of Defense

The nutrition label is your ally. Learning to interpret it accurately can mean the difference between a meal that stabilizes your blood sugar and one that derails your progress. Here's how to break it down:

- **Serving Size:** Always check this first. All nutritional information is based on this amount; eating more means multiplying the listed numbers.
- **Total Carbohydrates:** This figure includes all carbs—fiber, sugar, and starches. For blood sugar management, focus on "total carbohydrates" and "dietary fiber."
- **Dietary Fiber:** Higher fiber content generally lowers a food's glycemic impact. Subtract fiber from total carbohydrates to estimate net carbs, a practical step for low-GI eating.

- **Sugars:** Both natural and added sugars are included. Prefer foods with little or no added sugar.
- **Ingredients List:** Ingredients are listed by quantity, from highest to lowest. Look for whole foods and avoid items where sugar, corn syrup, or refined grains appear at the top.

Example:

Consider two breakfast cereals. The first lists whole grain oats, nuts, and dried fruit as its top ingredients, with 5g fiber, 7g sugars, and 35g total carbs per serving. The second lists corn syrup, puffed rice, and "natural flavors," with 1g fiber, 16g sugars, and 42g total carbs. The first cereal's higher fiber and lower sugar point to a better GI/GL profile.

Spotting Hidden Sugars and Unmasking GI Traps

Manufacturers are adept at disguising sugars under different names—**maltose, dextrose, honey, brown rice syrup**, and more. Even foods labeled as "natural" or "healthy" can harbor high-GI ingredients. Yogurts, salad dressings, and even savory snacks may contain surprising amounts of added sugars or refined starches.

Scan for multiple forms of sugar in the ingredient list.
Beware of "low-fat" claims; these often compensate for taste with extra sugar.
Watch out for "whole grain" products that are not 100% whole grain—read the label to confirm.

Using GI/GL in Everyday Shopping

Armed with GI and GL knowledge, you can make smarter swaps and plan meals that keep your blood glucose stable.

- **Choose whole foods:** Minimize packaged items where possible. Fresh vegetables, whole fruits, legumes, nuts, and whole grains are naturally low-GI.
- **Opt for minimally processed grains:** Brown rice, quinoa, barley, and oats have a gentler impact than white rice or refined flour.
- **Pair carbs with protein and healthy fat:** This slows digestion and reduces blood sugar spikes. For example, spread avocado or nut butter on whole grain toast instead of jam.
- **Consider portion size:** Even a low-GI food can raise blood sugar if eaten in large amounts. GI measures quality, while GL combines quality and quantity.

Global Perspective:

In Japan, the shift from a traditional diet of fish, vegetables, and moderate rice portions to Westernized, processed foods has paralleled rising rates of type 2 diabetes. Public health campaigns now encourage label reading and a return to whole ingredients, underscoring the global relevance of these skills.

Building Confidence: Practice Makes Progress

Like learning a new language, mastering food labels and GI/GL takes practice. Start with familiar foods and gradually expand your repertoire. Over time, you'll develop an intuitive sense of which products support your goals and which to leave on the shelf.

- Make a shopping list based on low-GI foods before you go.
- Compare two similar products for fiber, sugar, and total carbs.
- Keep a food journal—note how your choices affect your energy and blood sugar.

Fact: Even foods marketed as "diabetic friendly" can have high glycemic loads. Checking labels for total carbs, fiber, and sugar is always essential.

By turning the simple act of reading a food label into a daily habit, you empower yourself to outsmart hidden sugars and GI traps. These small, informed choices accumulate, transforming your meals and, ultimately, your health. In the next section, we'll assemble a practical GI/GL toolkit—recipes, swaps, and strategies to seamlessly integrate these principles into your day-to-day life, meal by meal. This is where knowledge becomes lasting change.

6.6 Case Studies in GI Success

From theory to practice, the glycemic index (GI) and glycemic load (GL) are more than numbers on a chart—they're tools that transform lives when put into action. Here, we turn to real-world stories and practical applications that illuminate how individuals around the globe have harnessed the power of GI and GL management to take control of their type 2 diabetes, often with remarkable results. These case studies offer inspiration, practical wisdom, and a reminder: sustainable change is not only possible, it's happening every day.

Maria's Mediterranean Makeover: A Journey of Small Swaps

Maria, a 58-year-old schoolteacher in southern Italy, was diagnosed with type 2 diabetes after years of enjoying refined breads and pastries so common in her region. Her physician introduced her to the concept of the glycemic index and encouraged a few changes—nothing drastic, just smarter choices within her beloved Mediterranean diet.

Maria's journey, chronicled in her own food diary and later shared in a national health magazine, is a testament to the power of incremental adjustments.

> She swapped white bread for whole-grain sourdough, reducing her breakfast GI. Fresh fruit replaced her mid-morning sweet pastry, providing fiber and micronutrients.
>
> Pasta, a staple in her home, was cooked al dente—lowering its GI, as less-cooked pasta is digested more slowly.
>
> Evening meals included legumes and leafy greens, which further moderated her blood glucose response.

Within three months, Maria's HbA1c—a measure of average blood sugar—dropped from 8.5% to 6.7%. She found her energy increasing, her mood improving, and her need for medication decreasing under her doctor's guidance. Maria's takeaway was simple: "I didn't give up the foods I loved; I just learned to love them in a new way."

The Singapore Solution: Community-Led Change

In Singapore, the government has long recognized the rising tide of type 2 diabetes, particularly among its fast-paced urban society. In 2016, a unique public health initiative known as the "War on Diabetes" was launched, focusing in part on GI education. The city-state's multicultural population—Chinese, Malay, Indian, and other groups—brought diverse food traditions and challenges.

> Local hawker centers introduced GI labeling on popular dishes, empowering diners to make informed choices.
>
> Public campaigns encouraged swapping high-GI staples like white rice for brown rice or mixed-grain alternatives.
>
> Cooking demonstrations in community centers showed how to prepare traditional favorites, such as nasi lemak and chicken rice, with lower-GI ingredients.

One striking example is Mr. Lim, a taxi driver who participated in a community program. By choosing brown rice and adding more non-starchy vegetables to his meals, he lost 10 kilograms and reduced his fasting glucose to prediabetic levels within six months. The initiative's success not only improved individual health outcomes but also fostered a sense of collective responsibility for diabetes prevention.

Lessons from Around the World

While Maria's story is one of personal adaptation and Singapore's is a testament to the power of public health policy, both underscore a universal truth: mastering GI and

GL is about context, culture, and creativity. Around the globe, people are finding ways to honor their heritage while embracing new strategies for blood sugar control.

In India, where white rice is a staple, nutritionists are working with families to incorporate more lentils, beans, and fiber-rich millets—foods that lower overall GL.

In Canada, Indigenous communities are reviving traditional diets rich in wild berries, fish, and root vegetables, many of which naturally have a low GI, supporting both cultural identity and metabolic health.

A Timeline of Change: How GI Awareness Spreads

Discovery: Researchers in the 1980s establish the glycemic index, linking carbohydrate quality to blood sugar response.

Adoption: Nutrition guidelines begin to incorporate GI/GL concepts in the 1990s and 2000s.

Personalization: Patients and clinicians today use GI/GL to tailor diets, with growing evidence for improved diabetes outcomes.

Globalization: Governments and communities worldwide implement GI education and food labeling, making change accessible at every level.

Maria and Mr. Lim's stories are not isolated successes; they reflect a broader movement toward informed, sustainable dietary choices. The science behind GI and GL may be universal, but its application is uniquely personal. By understanding the "why" and the "how," individuals can reclaim agency over their health, one meal at a time.

```
Did you know? Cooking pasta al dente can lower its glycemic index by up to 15
points compared to overcooked versions—helping steady your blood sugar!
```

```
Very important: Combining high-GI foods with healthy fats, proteins, or fiber
slows glucose absorption, reducing blood sugar spikes.
```

As we move forward, we'll translate these insights into your own daily life. In the next section, you'll find a hands-on GI/GL toolkit—recipes, food swaps, and everyday strategies—to help you put theory into practice. Because the most powerful change is the one you can sustain, meal after meal, year after year.

7 : Plant Power – Vegetarian & Plant-Based Strategies for Diabetes

7.1 The Science Behind Plant-Based Diets

Plant-based diets have surged in popularity worldwide—not just as a lifestyle choice or ethical stance, but as a powerful tool in the fight against type 2 diabetes. For many, the idea that what sits on our plate could dramatically influence blood sugar control and overall health is both empowering and, at times, overwhelming. Yet, the science is compelling: plant-based and vegetarian eating patterns can transform how our bodies manage glucose, reduce inflammation, and even reverse the course of diabetes.

The Core Principles of Plant-Based Nutrition

At its heart, a **plant-based diet** emphasizes vegetables, fruits, whole grains, legumes, nuts, and seeds, minimizing or excluding animal products. This approach offers a nutritional profile rich in fiber, antioxidants, vitamins, and minerals—nutrients that play crucial roles in metabolic health.

Several key principles underlie the diabetes-fighting power of plant-based diets:

Unveiling the Diabetes-Fighting Power of Plant-Based Diets

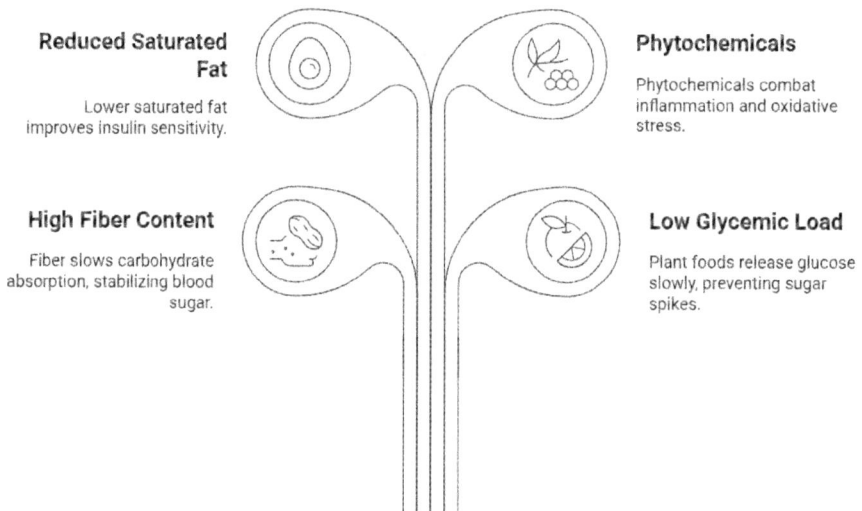

Reduced Saturated Fat — Lower saturated fat improves insulin sensitivity.

Phytochemicals — Phytochemicals combat inflammation and oxidative stress.

High Fiber Content — Fiber slows carbohydrate absorption, stabilizing blood sugar.

Low Glycemic Load — Plant foods release glucose slowly, preventing sugar spikes.

- **High fiber content:** Dietary fiber, especially soluble fiber found in beans, oats, and some fruits, slows carbohydrate absorption, blunting spikes in blood sugar.

- **Low glycemic load:** Many plant foods release glucose slowly, preventing rapid surges in blood sugar.
- **Reduced saturated fat:** Plant-based diets typically contain less saturated fat, which is linked to improved insulin sensitivity.
- **Phytochemicals:** Compounds like polyphenols, found in berries, leafy greens, and legumes, combat inflammation and oxidative stress, both of which are elevated in diabetes.

Evidence from the Field: Studies and Success Stories

Scientific research repeatedly highlights the benefits of plant-based diets for preventing and managing type 2 diabetes. In 2017, a landmark study published in the journal *Nutrients* reviewed data from over 200,000 adults and found that those following a predominantly plant-based diet had a 34% lower risk of developing type 2 diabetes.

But the impact goes beyond prevention. **Dr. Neal Barnard**, a pioneering researcher, conducted a randomized controlled trial comparing a low-fat vegan diet to a conventional diabetes diet. After 22 weeks, participants on the vegan diet experienced greater improvements in blood sugar control and, notably, some were able to reduce or eliminate their diabetes medications altogether.

Real-World Example: The Okinawan Experience

Okinawa, Japan, offers a living example of the power of plant-based eating. Traditionally, Okinawans consumed a diet based on sweet potatoes, vegetables, tofu, and minimal animal protein. For decades, rates of type 2 diabetes in Okinawa were among the lowest in the world. As Western dietary patterns infiltrated, diabetes rates climbed—a vivid reminder of the protective effect of plant-based nutrition.

How Plant-Based Diets Influence Diabetes at the Cellular Level

At the cellular level, plant-based diets promote **insulin sensitivity**. Insulin is the hormone that helps cells absorb glucose; in type 2 diabetes, cells become resistant to insulin's signal. Diets high in saturated fat and low in fiber exacerbate this resistance. Plant-based diets, by contrast, reduce fat buildup in muscle and liver cells, allowing insulin to work more effectively.

A plant-rich diet also improves **gut microbiota**—the vast community of microbes living in our digestive tract. These microbes ferment dietary fiber into short-chain fatty acids, which not only improve gut health but also enhance insulin sensitivity and reduce inflammation.

Cultural Variations: Global Approaches to Plant-Based Eating

Across the world, plant-based diets are woven into the fabric of traditional cuisines:

India: Many Indians practice vegetarianism, relying on lentils, chickpeas, and vegetables. These staples, rich in fiber and resistant starch, support steady blood sugar levels.

Mediterranean region: Here, meals center on grains, legumes, olives, and fresh produce. The Mediterranean diet, with its emphasis on plants and healthy fats, is associated with lower diabetes risk and improved metabolic health.

These global perspectives offer a wealth of ideas and ingredients for anyone seeking to manage diabetes through plant-based eating—reminding us that this approach is not a trend, but a time-honored tradition.

```
A high-fiber, plant-based diet can lower hemoglobin A1c levels as effectively
as some oral diabetes medications.
Switching to a plant-based diet has been shown in clinical trials to improve
insulin sensitivity within just a few weeks.
```

The science is clear: plant-based diets offer a potent, evidence-based strategy for reversing type 2 diabetes and reclaiming health. Whether rooted in cultural tradition or motivated by personal transformation, embracing plant power can bring rapid, lasting improvements in blood sugar control. Next, we'll translate this scientific foundation into practical steps—guiding you through meal planning, balanced nutrition, and easy, delicious recipes designed specifically for diabetes management.

7.2 Key Nutrients for Plant-Based Eaters

Transitioning to a plant-based or vegetarian lifestyle can be a powerful tool in the journey to reverse type 2 diabetes, but it does pose unique nutritional challenges. Unlike omnivorous diets, plant-based eating patterns require thoughtful planning to ensure all essential nutrients are consumed in the right amounts. The good news? With awareness and intention, vegetarian and vegan diets can not only meet but often exceed nutritional needs—fueling your body for optimal blood sugar control and long-term health.

The Six Essential Nutrients for Plant-Based Eaters

Let's explore the core nutrients every plant-based eater should prioritize for effective diabetes management:

- **Protein:** Crucial for muscle maintenance, satiety, and stable blood sugar.

- **Iron:** Supports energy and oxygen transport, especially vital for those who avoid red meat.
- **Vitamin B12:** Essential for nerve function and red blood cell formation, generally lacking in plant foods.
- **Omega-3 Fatty Acids:** Support heart health and reduce inflammation, particularly important for people with diabetes.
- **Calcium:** Vital for bone strength and metabolic health.
- **Vitamin D:** Supports immune function and calcium absorption.

Essential Nutrients for Plant-Based Diabetes Management

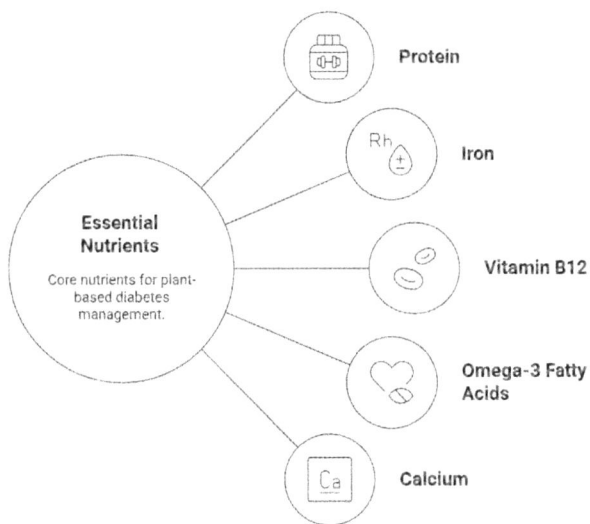

Each of these nutrients plays a distinct role in the body's intricate metabolic processes, and missing even one can impact your progress toward reversing type 2 diabetes.

Protein: Building Blocks for Blood Sugar Balance

Plant-based sources of protein include beans, lentils, tofu, tempeh, soy milk, quinoa, nuts, and seeds. While animal proteins are "complete," meaning they contain all nine essential amino acids, most plant proteins are "incomplete." However, by eating a diverse mix of plant foods throughout the day, you can easily achieve complete protein intake.

Iron: Preventing Deficiency and Supporting Energy

Iron is abundant in plant foods like lentils, spinach, chickpeas, tofu, and fortified cereals. However, plant-based iron (non-heme iron) is less readily absorbed by the body.

To enhance absorption, combine iron-rich foods with vitamin C sources, such as tomatoes, bell peppers, or citrus fruits.

- Add lemon juice to spinach salads.
- Pair bean chili with a side of fresh oranges.
- Include tomatoes in lentil soups.

Vitamin B12: The Non-Negotiable Supplement

Vitamin B12 is one of the few nutrients not naturally present in plant foods. Deficiency can lead to fatigue, nerve damage, and impaired cognitive function—symptoms that can mask or worsen diabetic complications. Regular supplementation or consuming fortified foods (like nutritional yeast or plant milks) is essential.

Omega-3 Fatty Acids: Plant-Based Sources for Heart Health

Omega-3s are vital for reducing inflammation and supporting cardiovascular health—a top priority for those managing diabetes. While fatty fish is a common source, vegetarians can turn to:

- Flaxseeds and flaxseed oil
- Chia seeds
- Walnuts
- Algal oil supplements (derived from algae)

These foods provide alpha-linolenic acid (ALA), a plant-based omega-3, which the body can convert—albeit inefficiently—into the longer-chain forms found in fish.

Calcium and Vitamin D: The Bone and Immune Protectors

Calcium is found in fortified plant milks, tofu set with calcium, leafy greens (like bok choy and kale), almonds, and sesame seeds. Vitamin D, on the other hand, is synthesized in the skin through sunlight exposure. In regions with little sunlight or for individuals with dark skin, fortified foods or supplements may be necessary.

- Check plant-based milks for added vitamin D and calcium.
- Spend a few minutes outdoors each day, or speak with your healthcare provider about supplementation.

A Global Perspective: Plant-Based Traditions and Diabetes

Around the world, plant-based eating has deep roots. In Ethiopia, injera (a sour flatbread made from teff) is paired with lentil stews, providing fiber and plant protein. In the Mediterranean, legumes and vegetables form the basis of daily meals, contributing to the region's notably low rates of chronic disease. These culinary traditions underline how plant-powered diets, when balanced, can foster lasting health and diabetes resilience.

```
Plant-based diets are associated with up to a 34% lower risk of developing
type 2 diabetes. Vitamin B12 is the one micronutrient virtually absent from
plant foods—supplementation is essential.
```

Putting It All Together

A thoughtful plant-based diet can deliver all the nutrients needed to manage and even reverse type 2 diabetes. By focusing on variety, planning for nutrient gaps, and drawing inspiration from global traditions, you can create meals that are not only delicious but powerfully therapeutic.

As we move forward, we'll bring these principles into your kitchen, sharing practical tips for meal planning, easy recipes, and strategies to navigate social and cultural challenges. You're building a toolkit not just for diabetes management, but for lifelong vitality—one meal at a time.

7.3 Building Balanced Plant-Based Meals

Designing meals as a vegetarian or plant-based eater with type 2 diabetes can seem like navigating a culinary puzzle. Yet, with a thoughtful approach, every plate becomes an opportunity to optimize blood sugar, enjoy delicious foods, and celebrate vibrant health. The essence lies in balance—combining macronutrients, selecting low-glycemic ingredients, and infusing meals with flavor and satisfaction.

The Foundation: Macronutrient Balance

A healthy plant-based meal for diabetes management is more than just eliminating animal products. It's about constructing each meal with the right proportions of the three key macronutrients: carbohydrates, proteins, and healthy fats.

Carbohydrates: Opt for whole, minimally processed sources such as lentils, chickpeas, beans, oats, quinoa, sweet potatoes, and whole grains. These foods offer fiber that slows glucose absorption, moderating post-meal blood sugar spikes.

Proteins: Incorporate plant-based proteins like tofu, tempeh, edamame, seitan, and legumes. These not only support satiety but also help maintain muscle mass, which is crucial for metabolic health.

Healthy Fats: Avocados, nuts, seeds, and olive oil provide essential fatty acids that support heart health and further stabilize glucose levels.

A simple guideline is the "plate method": fill half your plate with non-starchy vegetables (like leafy greens, peppers, or broccoli), one quarter with whole grains or starchy vegetables, and one quarter with plant proteins. Add a drizzle of healthy fats or a handful of nuts for flavor and nourishment.

Low-Glycemic Choices: Eating for Gentle Blood Sugar Rises

Understanding the **glycemic index (GI)** and **glycemic load (GL)** is vital in crafting meals. Choose foods that release glucose slowly, keeping blood sugar steady.

Low-GI foods: Lentils, beans, non-starchy vegetables, steel-cut oats, barley, and most fruits like berries and apples.

Medium-GI foods: Brown rice, sweet potatoes, pineapple, and whole wheat bread.

High-GI foods (use sparingly): White bread, most breakfast cereals, white rice, and potatoes.

Pairing carbohydrates with fiber, protein, or fat further lowers a meal's overall glycemic impact. For example, topping steel-cut oats with chia seeds and berries, or pairing hummus with whole grain pita and sliced cucumbers, creates a synergistic effect.

Crafting a Day of Balanced Plant-Based Meals

Let's walk through a sample day:

- **Breakfast:** Overnight oats made with rolled oats, unsweetened almond milk, chia seeds, and blueberries. A sprinkle of walnuts adds crunch and healthy fat.
- **Lunch:** Quinoa and black bean salad with a rainbow of chopped vegetables, tossed in olive oil and lemon. Add a side of roasted Brussels sprouts for fiber.
- **Snack:** Sliced apple with almond butter, or carrot sticks with hummus.
- **Dinner:** Stir-fried tofu with broccoli, bell peppers, and snap peas, served over brown rice. Top with sesame seeds for extra nutrition.

What should I eat for a balanced plant-based meal?

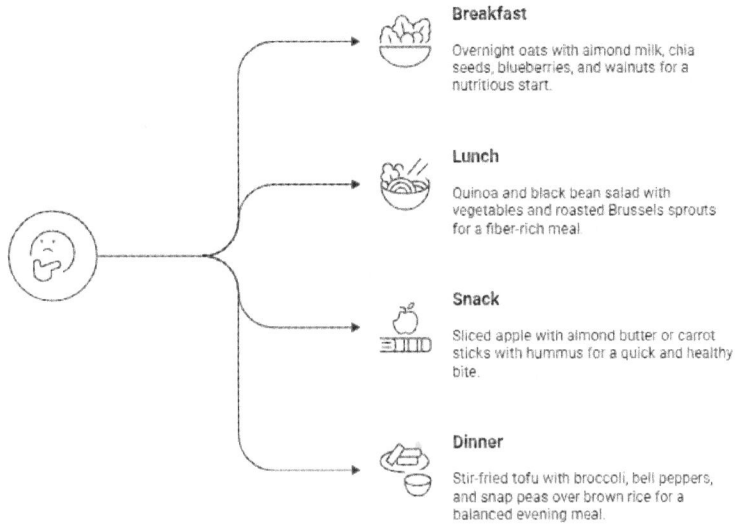

Breakfast

Overnight oats with almond milk, chia seeds, blueberries, and walnuts for a nutritious start.

Lunch

Quinoa and black bean salad with vegetables and roasted Brussels sprouts for a fiber-rich meal.

Snack

Sliced apple with almond butter or carrot sticks with hummus for a quick and healthy bite.

Dinner

Stir-fried tofu with broccoli, bell peppers, and snap peas over brown rice for a balanced evening meal.

By choosing a variety of colors and textures, you not only make meals more appealing but also ensure a diversity of nutrients.

Meal Planning for Social and Cultural Joy

Plant-based eating doesn't mean sacrificing tradition or flavor. Whether it's a family gathering or a festive holiday, focus on adapting recipes rather than avoiding them. For instance, swap out white rice for cauliflower rice in biryani, or use mashed white beans and herbs in place of cheese spreads for appetizers. Share your journey with friends and family—often, they'll be curious and supportive, and may even join you in trying new dishes.

Quick Reference: Memorable Tips

```
- Fiber is your friend: Aim for at least 25-30 grams per day from whole foods.
- Pair carbs with protein/fat for steady blood sugar.
```

Building balanced plant-based meals is both a science and an art, rooted in simple principles yet rich with cultural and personal expression. By mastering these strategies, you not only support your diabetes reversal journey but also rediscover the pleasure of nourishing, flavorful food. Up next, we'll explore how to navigate eating out, special occasions, and social situations with confidence—ensuring your path to lasting health is as joyful as it is sustainable.

7.4 Cultural Plant-Based Diets

Across continents and centuries, plant-based diets have long been woven into the fabric of many cultures—offering not just sustenance, but a framework for health, community, and tradition. As we embrace plant-powered strategies for managing type 2 diabetes, exploring these time-honored dietary patterns can offer both inspiring models and practical tools for real-world success.

The Roots of Plant-Based Traditions

Many of the world's most celebrated plant-based diets emerged not from modern health trends, but from ancestral wisdom shaped by geography, climate, and spirituality. These traditions have thrived across generations, often supporting vibrant health and remarkable longevity.

- **The Mediterranean Diet**: Encompassing countries like Greece, Italy, and southern Spain, this diet is rich in vegetables, legumes, whole grains, fruits, nuts, and olive oil—with only modest portions of fish and dairy. Research consistently links the Mediterranean pattern to lower rates of type 2 diabetes, heart disease, and obesity.
- **Traditional South Asian Diets**: In regions of India, Nepal, and Sri Lanka, vegetarianism is deeply rooted in religious and cultural values. Meals typically revolve around lentils, beans, rice, whole grains, vegetables, spices, and ghee or plant oils. Notably, the fiber and phytonutrient content of these diets aid in stabilizing blood sugar and promoting digestive health.
- **East Asian Plant-Centric Eating**: In places like rural China, Japan, and Korea, daily meals historically feature seasonal vegetables, soy products (such as tofu and tempeh), fermented foods, and rice. Animal protein is used in small amounts, often as a flavor accent rather than the main attraction.

Adapting Cultural Diets for Modern Diabetes Care

Modern lifestyles often pull us away from these nourishing traditions, but their wisdom is more relevant than ever. For individuals managing diabetes, returning to—or adapting—these plant-based patterns can offer a blueprint for lasting health. Consider these practical adaptations:

- Swap white rice for brown rice or quinoa to increase fiber and lower the glycemic load.
- Emphasize legumes and lentils as protein sources, cutting back on processed meats.

- Use herbs and spices (like turmeric, cumin, and basil) for flavor, which may also offer anti-inflammatory benefits.
- Incorporate fermented foods, such as kimchi, miso, or yogurt, to support gut health—a crucial component of metabolic wellness.

Global Insights on Plant-Based Patterns

While each culture's plant-based traditions are unique, they share important features that support diabetes reversal:

- Emphasis on whole, minimally processed ingredients
- Use of plant proteins (beans, lentils, soy) as staples
- Balanced meals with healthy fats, complex carbs, and micronutrients
- Portion awareness and mindful eating practices

Across the globe, from Ethiopian injera with lentil stews to Mexican black bean tacos, these foods nourish both body and spirit—proving that healthful eating can be deeply satisfying and culturally meaningful.

Key Takeaways for Your Own Plate

- Look to your cultural heritage for inspiration—reviving traditional dishes can make healthy eating more enjoyable and sustainable.
- Don't be afraid to blend customs—fusion meals can draw from multiple plant-based traditions to create new favorites.
- Remember: it's not just what you eat, but how you eat—sharing meals, practicing gratitude, and eating mindfully are all part of the healing process.

```
Fact: Diets high in whole, plant-based foods and low in refined carbohydrates
have been shown to improve insulin sensitivity and may help reverse type 2
diabetes in as little as 12 weeks.
```

As you move forward, let these cultural plant-based diets inspire your own journey. Next, we'll tackle the real-world challenges of eating out, handling special occasions, and thriving in social settings—equipping you with strategies to maintain your progress wherever life takes you. By honoring both tradition and innovation, you can craft a path to diabetes reversal that is as nourishing for the soul as it is for the body.

7.5 Overcoming Common Challenges

Navigating a plant-based approach to diabetes management brings unique benefits, but it also comes with its own set of hurdles. As you embark on this path, it's normal to encounter challenges—both practical and psychological. The good news: with understanding and preparation, these obstacles can become stepping stones toward lasting health.

Protein: Meeting Needs Without Meat

A common concern among those new to vegetarian or vegan diets is **getting enough protein**. The myth that animal products are the only reliable protein source remains persistent, yet history and modern evidence reveal otherwise. For example, the traditional diets of South Indian communities—rich in lentils, chickpeas, and fermented legumes—have nourished generations while supporting stable blood sugar levels.

- **Plant-based protein sources**: Beans, lentils, tofu, tempeh, edamame, seitan, quinoa, nuts, and seeds.
- **Combining proteins**: While most plant proteins are "incomplete," diverse daily intake ensures all essential amino acids are met.
- **Portion awareness**: Since plant proteins may be less calorie-dense, larger or more frequent servings might be required.

One inspiring story is that of **Asha**, a grandmother from Mumbai, who reversed her type 2 diabetes markers by swapping out white rice for sprouted lentils and millet, all while maintaining her vegetarian traditions. Her story reminds us that dietary shifts don't require abandoning cultural identity—they can, in fact, deepen it.

Carbohydrates: Navigating the Glycemic Maze

Plant-based diets tend to be higher in carbohydrates, which can be daunting for those managing blood sugar. But not all carbs are created equal. Understanding **glycemic index (GI)** and **glycemic load (GL)** is crucial:

Low-GI choices: Legumes, most vegetables, whole grains like barley or steel-cut oats.

Smart swaps: Replace white rice with quinoa or brown rice; choose whole fruit over juice.

Fiber focus: High-fiber foods slow glucose absorption, blunting blood sugar spikes.

A historical example comes from Okinawa, Japan, where centenarians traditionally consumed sweet potatoes—a low-GI, high-fiber staple. Their longevity and low rates of diabetes highlight the importance of **quality over quantity** when it comes to carbohydrates.

Social and Cultural Pressures

Food is often at the heart of community and family life. Navigating social gatherings, religious holidays, or travel can present temptations and barriers:

- **Plan ahead**: Offer to bring a plant-based dish to share.
- **Communicate**: Explain your choices to friends and family, inviting their support.
- **Practice flexibility**: If options are limited, focus on portion control and balance.

Consider **Carlos**, a Mexican-American father living in Los Angeles, who found it challenging to attend family fiestas without indulging in traditional, meat-heavy dishes. He gradually introduced black bean tamales and vegetable pozole to family events, eventually inspiring others to join his journey toward better health.

Micronutrient Pitfalls

While plant-based diets are rich in many vitamins and minerals, certain nutrients require extra attention:

- **Vitamin B12**: Not naturally found in plants; supplementing is essential for vegans.
- **Iron**: Plant-based iron (non-heme) is less easily absorbed; pair with vitamin C-rich foods.
- **Omega-3 fatty acids**: Flaxseeds, chia seeds, walnuts, and algae-based supplements provide plant sources.

Routine blood work and consultation with healthcare providers help ensure that your nutritional bases are covered.

Overcoming Cravings and Emotional Eating

Shifting to a new way of eating can stir up cravings, especially for processed foods or old favorites. Emotional eating, often triggered by stress, boredom, or celebration, can derail progress. Strategies include:

- **Mindful eating**: Pay attention to hunger and fullness cues.
- **Healthy swaps**: Prepare plant-based versions of comfort foods, like lentil shepherd's pie or black bean brownies.
- **Stress management**: Incorporate practices like yoga, meditation, or walking.

Practical Tips for Daily Success

- **Meal prep**: Batch-cook grains, beans, and vegetables to simplify weeknight meals.
- **Pack snacks**: Keep nuts, seeds, or roasted chickpeas on hand to avoid vending machine pitfalls.
- **Stay informed**: Continue learning about nutrition, recipes, and cultural adaptations.

Building a Support System

Surrounding yourself with like-minded individuals can make all the difference:

- **Local groups**: Seek out vegetarian meetups, diabetes support circles, or cooking classes.
- **Online communities**: Join forums or social media groups for recipe ideas and encouragement.

Remember, you are not alone on this journey. Across continents and cultures, individuals are embracing plant-based living to reclaim their health.

```
A well-planned vegetarian or plant-based diet can provide all the nutrients
required for reversing type 2 diabetes—just be mindful of B12 and iron!
```

In summary, overcoming common challenges on a plant-based path to diabetes reversal is entirely achievable with knowledge, planning, and support. By honoring your heritage, embracing new traditions, and staying proactive, you can transform obstacles into opportunities for healing. As you move forward, the next section explores how to integrate exercise and movement into your daily routine—an essential companion to lasting dietary change.

7.6 Sample Menus and Recipes

Embracing a vegetarian or plant-based approach to managing type 2 diabetes doesn't mean settling for bland or repetitive meals. Instead, it opens a world of colorful, nutritionally dense foods that both nourish and delight. The real secret lies in creating balanced meals that optimize blood sugar control while satisfying your palate. This section provides sample daily menus and a handful of recipes, all rooted in glycemic index (GI) awareness and tailored to meet the unique needs of individuals managing diabetes.

Principles Behind the Menus

Each menu below is thoughtfully crafted to:

- Prioritize **low-GI and low-glycemic-load foods** to promote stable blood sugar.

- Include a balance of **complex carbohydrates**, **lean plant-based proteins**, and **healthy fats**.
- Incorporate a variety of **fiber-rich vegetables** and **whole grains**.
- Limit processed foods, added sugars, and refined starches.

To truly succeed, flexibility is key—these menus are guides, not rigid prescriptions. Adjust portions and swap ingredients based on availability, seasonality, and personal preferences.

A Day on Your Plate: Sample Menu

Let's walk through a sample day that demonstrates how easy—and enjoyable—plant-powered eating can be.

- **Breakfast:**

  - **Overnight Chia Pudding**: Soak 3 tablespoons of chia seeds in unsweetened almond milk with a dash of cinnamon and a handful of fresh berries.
  - **Herbal tea** or black coffee (no sugar added).

  - **Mid-Morning Snack:**

  - **Apple slices** with 1 tablespoon natural almond butter.

- **Lunch:**

  - **Quinoa & Chickpea Salad**: Toss cooked quinoa with chickpeas, diced cucumber, cherry tomatoes, chopped parsley, and a lemon-tahini dressing.
  - **Steamed broccoli** on the side.

  - **Afternoon Snack:**

  - **Carrot sticks** and hummus.

- **Dinner:**

  - **Lentil & Spinach Stew**: Simmer green lentils with onions, garlic, diced tomatoes, and baby spinach, seasoned with cumin and coriander.
  - **Side of roasted cauliflower**.

  - **Dessert (optional):**

o **Sliced kiwi** or a few cubes of fresh papaya.

Recipes to Jumpstart Your Journey

Let's bring these ideas to life with a few favorite recipes that balance flavor and blood sugar management.

Lentil & Spinach Stew

Serves 4

- 1 cup dry green or brown lentils, rinsed
- 1 medium onion, chopped
- 2 garlic cloves, minced
- 1 can (14 oz) diced tomatoes (no sugar added)
- 4 cups vegetable broth (low sodium)
- 2 cups fresh spinach
- 1 teaspoon ground cumin
- 1/2 teaspoon ground coriander
- Salt and pepper to taste
- 1 tablespoon olive oil

Preparation

- In a large pot, heat olive oil over medium heat. Add onion and cook until translucent.
- Stir in garlic, cumin, and coriander; cook for 1 minute.
- Add lentils, diced tomatoes, and vegetable broth. Bring to a boil, then reduce heat and simmer uncovered for 25-30 minutes, or until lentils are tender.
- Stir in spinach and cook until wilted. Season with salt and pepper to taste.
- Serve hot, garnished with fresh herbs if desired.

Quinoa & Chickpea Salad

Serves 2

- 1 cup cooked quinoa
- 1/2 cup cooked or canned chickpeas, rinsed and drained
- 1/2 cucumber, diced
- 1/2 cup cherry tomatoes, halved
- 1/4 cup chopped parsley

- Juice of 1 lemon
- 2 tablespoons tahini
- 1 tablespoon olive oil
- Salt and pepper to taste

Preparation

- In a large bowl, combine quinoa, chickpeas, cucumber, tomatoes, and parsley.
- In a small bowl, whisk together lemon juice, tahini, olive oil, salt, and pepper.
- Pour dressing over salad and toss to combine.
- Chill before serving for best flavor.

Historical Perspective: The Mediterranean Connection

The Mediterranean diet, rich in legumes, whole grains, vegetables, and olive oil, has long garnered attention for its diabetes-fighting potential. Studies from Greece, Italy, and Spain reveal that those following plant-forward Mediterranean patterns often experience lower rates of type 2 diabetes and cardiovascular disease. This historical approach, emphasizing seasonal produce and simple preparations, aligns beautifully with modern plant-based diabetes care.

Tips for Cultural Adaptation

No matter where you live, plant-based diabetes management can be tailored to local tastes:

- In **Latin America**, try black bean and vegetable tacos with corn tortillas (choose whole corn) and avocado salsa.
- In **East Asia**, savor stir-fried tofu with bok choy, shiitake mushrooms, and brown rice.
- In **West Africa**, enjoy a groundnut stew with lentils, leafy greens, and tomatoes over fonio or millet.

```
- Fiber from legumes and whole grains slows glucose absorption, reducing blood
sugar spikes.
- Plant-based diets can significantly improve insulin sensitivity and reduce
medication needs in type 2 diabetes.
```

Embracing plant-powered eating for diabetes is as much about pleasure as it is about health. With a little creativity and an open mind, every meal becomes an opportunity for healing. These menus and recipes are just the beginning—personalize them to your tastes and culture, and you'll discover that nourishing your body can be both simple and satisfying.

As we move forward, the next chapter will explore the vital role of movement. Exercise, when paired with smart nutrition, amplifies your body's ability to reverse type 2 diabetes—turning small daily decisions into lifelong health. Let's step into the world of activity and discover how movement can be your ally on this journey.

8 : Movement Matters – Exercise and Physical Activity for Reversal

8.1 Why Exercise Works for Diabetes

Imagine a medicine so powerful it could regulate your blood sugar, lower your risk for heart disease, and lift your mood—all without a prescription or side effects. This "medicine" exists, and it's called **exercise**. For those aiming to reverse type 2 diabetes, movement isn't just an optional add-on; it's a cornerstone of lasting health.

The Science: How Exercise Affects Blood Sugar

To understand why exercise works for diabetes, we need to peek beneath the surface of the body's biology. In type 2 diabetes, the body's cells become resistant to **insulin**, the hormone responsible for moving glucose out of the bloodstream and into cells for energy. This leads to high blood sugar, which, over time, damages organs and blood vessels.

Exercise tackles this problem in several remarkable ways:

Exercise's Impact on Insulin Sensitivity

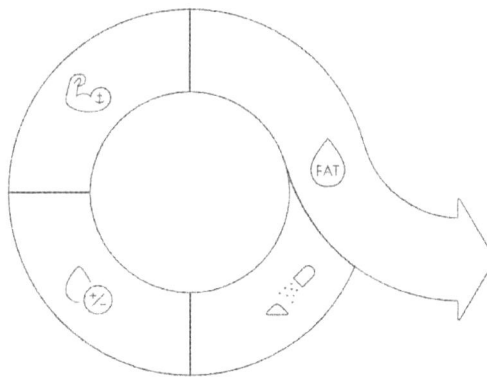

1	2	3	4
Increase Insulin Sensitivity	**Reduce Blood Sugar**	**Build Muscle Mass**	**Enhance Fat Metabolism**
Muscles become more receptive to insulin.	Muscles use glucose for energy.	Larger glucose storage capacity.	Reduces circulating fat levels.

- **Increases Insulin Sensitivity**: When you move your muscles, they become more receptive to insulin—almost like opening more doors for sugar to enter.
- **Reduces Blood Sugar Immediately**: Muscles use glucose for energy during activity, lowering your blood sugar even if insulin is not working perfectly.
- **Builds Muscle Mass**: More muscle means a larger "storage tank" for glucose, helping to stabilize blood sugar levels over the long term.
- **Enhances Fat Metabolism**: Regular activity helps reduce the amount of circulating fat in the bloodstream, which is linked to improved insulin action.

Research has shown that even a single session of moderate exercise can improve insulin sensitivity for the next 24–48 hours—a testament to its immediate power.

A Tale from History: From Ancient Healing to Modern Science

Physical movement has long been recognized as a pillar of health. Ancient Greek physician **Hippocrates** advised his patients to combine "the right amount of food and exercise" to maintain health. Fast-forward to the 20th century, before modern diabetes medications were widely available, and doctors would often send newly diagnosed diabetes patients on long walks as a first-line treatment. While our scientific understanding has advanced, the wisdom of movement remains as relevant as ever.

Why Exercise Delivers Unique Benefits for Diabetes

Exercise stands apart from other interventions for several reasons:

- **Works Independently of Weight Loss**: Even if the scale doesn't budge, exercise still boosts insulin sensitivity and lowers blood sugar.
- **Reduces Medication Needs**: Many people find they can decrease or even stop certain diabetes medications as their activity level rises (always in consultation with their doctor).
- **Protects Heart Health**: Given that people with diabetes are at increased risk for heart disease, the cardiovascular benefits of exercise are especially vital.
- **Improves Mental Well-Being**: Physical activity releases endorphins, helping to combat the anxiety and depression that sometimes accompany chronic illness.

Exercise Benefits Cycle for Diabetes

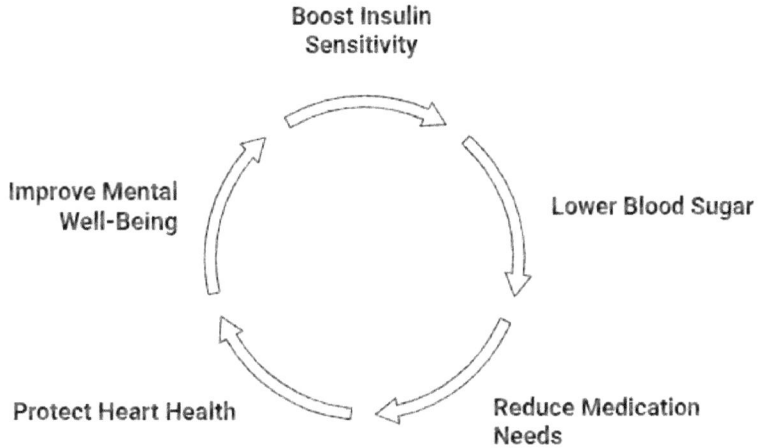

Boost Insulin
Sensitivity

Lower Blood Sugar

Reduce Medication
Needs

Protect Heart Health

Improve Mental
Well-Being

Types of Exercise: Finding What Fits

Not all movement is created equal, but the good news is that almost any form of activity helps. The most effective routines combine:

The Power of Combined Movement Routines

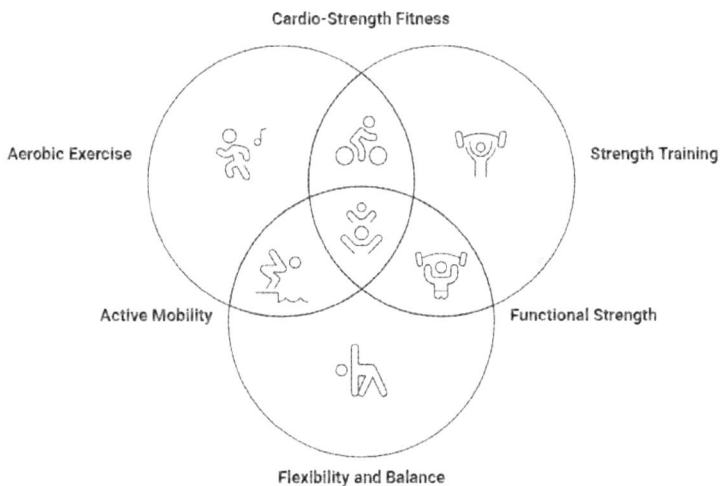

Cardio-Strength Fitness

Aerobic Exercise

Strength Training

Active Mobility

Functional Strength

Flexibility and Balance

- **Aerobic Exercise** (walking, cycling, swimming): Great for overall cardiovascular health and immediate blood sugar reduction.
- **Strength Training** (weight lifting, resistance bands, bodyweight exercises): Crucial for building and maintaining muscle mass.
- **Flexibility and Balance** (yoga, tai chi): Support joint health and can reduce the risk of falls, especially in older adults.

Global Perspectives: Movement Across Cultures

Different cultures have embraced movement as medicine in diverse ways. In **Japan**, daily group exercises called **rajio taisō** (radio calisthenics) are broadcast throughout the country, promoting lifelong habits of activity. In India, yoga is not just a spiritual practice but a therapeutic tool for managing diabetes and other chronic conditions. These examples show that movement can be woven into daily life in ways that are joyful, social, and sustainable.

How Quickly Does Exercise Make a Difference?

The timeline for seeing benefits can be surprisingly fast:

- **Within Hours**: Blood sugar levels may drop after just one session.
- **Within Weeks**: Insulin sensitivity improves, and energy levels rise.
- **Within Months**: Weight loss, lower cholesterol, and reduced need for medication become evident.

The key is consistency, not intensity—regular, moderate activity is often more effective (and sustainable) than sporadic bursts of hard exercise.

Fact: Just 150 minutes per week of moderate exercise—such as brisk walking—can significantly reduce blood sugar and the risk of diabetes complications.

Exercise is more than a tool for managing diabetes; it's a catalyst for transformation, empowering you to take charge of your health, one step at a time. Whether your path is a daily stroll, a yoga practice, or joining a dance class, the science is clear: movement matters.

As we turn to the next section, we'll explore how to create a realistic and enjoyable exercise routine—one that fits your lifestyle, respects your body, and fuels your journey toward lasting health and diabetes reversal.

8.2 Types of Physical Activity

When it comes to reversing type 2 diabetes, not all movement is created equal. The body responds differently to various forms of physical activity, and understanding these distinctions helps tailor an approach that maximizes both enjoyment and results.

Let's explore the main categories of physical activity that empower individuals in their journey toward diabetes reversal.

1. Aerobic (Cardio) Exercise

Aerobic activity, often called "cardio," gets your heart pumping and increases the circulation of oxygen throughout your body. This form of exercise is especially effective at lowering blood glucose levels and improving insulin sensitivity.

> **Examples:** Brisk walking, cycling, swimming, jogging, dancing, and even energetic gardening.
>
> **How it works:** Muscles use glucose (blood sugar) for energy, drawing it from the bloodstream and leading to lower resting blood sugar levels post-exercise.
>
> **Recommended duration:** The American Diabetes Association suggests at least 150 minutes of moderate-intensity aerobic activity per week, spread across most days.
>
> **Real-World Example:**

In the bustling streets of Copenhagen, Denmark, cycling is more than a pastime—it's a way of life. Adults of all ages commute by bike, rain or shine. Studies from Denmark have shown that regular cycling is associated with a significantly reduced risk of developing type 2 diabetes. For those already diagnosed, adopting cycling—whether outdoors or on a stationary bike—has yielded consistent improvements in blood sugar control and cardiovascular health.

2. Resistance (Strength) Training

Building muscle isn't just for athletes. **Resistance training**—using weights, resistance bands, or your own body weight—offers profound benefits for those managing or reversing type 2 diabetes.

> **Examples:** Lifting weights, using resistance bands, bodyweight exercises like squats or push-ups, Pilates, and certain forms of yoga.
>
> **How it works:** Muscle tissue is a primary site for glucose uptake. The more muscle you have, the more efficiently your body can clear glucose from the bloodstream.
>
> **Frequency:** Aim for two to three sessions per week, targeting all major muscle groups.
>
> **Personal Story:**

Meet Maria, a 58-year-old retiree from Mexico City. After her type 2 diabetes diagnosis, traditional walking routines yielded only modest improvements. It wasn't until she joined a local women's fitness club and started circuit training with light weights that her blood sugar readings began to normalize. Maria's story illustrates that strength training can be transformative, especially for those who may not initially consider themselves "fitness types."

3. Flexibility and Balance Exercises

While these activities may seem less intense, they play a pivotal role in a well-rounded routine—especially for older adults or those with mobility challenges.

Examples: Yoga, Tai Chi, stretching routines, balance drills.

How it works: Enhances joint mobility, reduces the risk of falls, and can ease muscle stiffness—making daily movement more accessible and enjoyable.

Unique benefits: Certain forms, like yoga and Tai Chi, also incorporate stress reduction and mindfulness, further supporting blood sugar management.

Global Perspective:

In China, the early-morning sight of people practicing Tai Chi in public parks is iconic. Clinical research has demonstrated that regular Tai Chi practice can lower fasting blood glucose and improve overall quality of life for people with type 2 diabetes.

4. Non-Exercise Physical Activity (NEPA)

Not all movement needs to be structured. **Non-Exercise Physical Activity** refers to the energy you expend in daily life outside of deliberate exercise.

Examples: Walking to the store, household chores, gardening, taking the stairs, playing with pets or children.

Why it matters: Small bursts of movement throughout the day can cumulatively lower blood sugar and counteract the negative effects of prolonged sitting.

Practical tip: Set a timer to stand and move every hour, or incorporate "walking meetings" into your workday.

5. High-Intensity Interval Training (HIIT)

For those looking for efficiency, **HIIT** involves alternating short bursts of intense activity with periods of rest or lower-intensity movement.

Examples: Sprinting followed by walking, cycling sprints, or interval circuits with bodyweight exercises.

How it works: HIIT is shown to rapidly improve insulin sensitivity and cardiovascular fitness with shorter time commitments.

Caution: Beginners or those with heart conditions should consult their healthcare provider before starting HIIT.

Making It Culturally Your Own

Movement takes many forms across cultures—traditional dances in India, community walks in South Africa, or group swimming in Australia. The key is to find activities aligned with your traditions, preferences, and social support systems. This not only increases adherence but brings joy to the journey.

```
Important: Just 30 minutes of moderate physical activity most days can
significantly lower your risk of diabetes complications and support reversal—
even if broken into smaller sessions throughout the day.
```

In summary, the types of physical activity available are as diverse as the people undertaking them. Whether you choose brisk walks, resistance bands, mindful yoga, or playful daily movement, each step moves you closer to lasting health. In the next section, we'll guide you through crafting a personalized exercise routine—one that fits your unique lifestyle, respects your physical abilities, and keeps you motivated on the path to reversing type 2 diabetes.

8.3 Building an Exercise Routine

Understanding Your Starting Point

Before you lace up your sneakers or unroll your yoga mat, it's crucial to begin with an honest assessment of your current physical condition. This self-inventory isn't about judgment—it's about safety and setting yourself up for success. Consider your age, weight, any physical limitations, past injuries, and your typical daily activity level. If you're managing other health conditions alongside type 2 diabetes, consult your healthcare provider to determine what types and intensities of exercise are appropriate for you.

For many, this initial step is empowering. Take the story of **Luis**, a 62-year-old retired teacher from Madrid, who hadn't exercised regularly in decades. After his diagnosis, he worked with his doctor to create a simple walking program. Over time, these regular strolls became brisk walks, then hikes with friends, and his blood sugar levels improved dramatically. Luis's experience highlights the importance of starting where you are and building momentum.

The Core Elements of an Effective Routine

An effective diabetes-reversal exercise regimen blends several types of physical activity. Each offers unique benefits for blood sugar control, cardiovascular health, and overall well-being.

Aerobic Exercise: Activities like brisk walking, swimming, cycling, or dancing raise your heart rate and burn calories, helping to increase insulin sensitivity.

Resistance Training: Lifting weights, using resistance bands, or bodyweight exercises (like squats and push-ups) build muscle mass, which enhances glucose uptake.

Flexibility and Balance: Yoga, tai chi, and stretching improve mobility, reduce injury risk, and can alleviate stress—a known contributor to high blood sugar.

A well-rounded weekly routine might include:

- 150 minutes of moderate-intensity aerobic activity
- Two sessions of resistance training
- Flexibility and balance exercises 2–3 times per week

But remember: even short bursts of movement count. Ten-minute walks after meals, gardening, or climbing stairs all contribute meaningfully to your progress.

Crafting a Sustainable Plan

Consistency, not perfection, is the foundation of lasting change. Let's outline a simple five-step process for building your personalized exercise routine:

- **Set Realistic Goals:** Start with achievable, measurable targets—like walking 10 minutes a day, three times a week.
- **Mix It Up:** Combine activities you enjoy to maintain interest and motivation. Variety also works different muscle groups and prevents plateaus.
- **Schedule It:** Block out time in your calendar, just as you would for a meeting or appointment. Consistency creates habit.
- **Track Your Progress:** Keep a simple log or use an app to monitor your activity, energy levels, and blood sugar readings. Celebrate small wins!
- **Adjust as Needed:** Listen to your body. If something isn't working—whether due to pain, boredom, or schedule—adapt your routine rather than abandoning it altogether.

Take inspiration from **Rashmi**, a 45-year-old office worker in Mumbai. She began her journey with daily stretches and weekend dance classes. Over months, she incorporated cycling and resistance band workouts, finding joy in variety and a support network in her local community center.

Overcoming Barriers and Staying Motivated

It's normal to encounter obstacles—busy schedules, fatigue, bad weather, or self-doubt. Here are practical strategies to keep moving forward:

- **Find an Accountability Partner:** Exercise with a friend, join a class, or engage with an online group for support.
- **Make it Enjoyable:** Listen to music, podcasts, or audiobooks to transform exercise into a pleasurable routine.
- **Embrace Cultural Practices:** In many cultures, group movement—such as African dance, Latin American Zumba, or Chinese tai chi—offers both physical benefits and social connection.
- **Be Kind to Yourself:** Progress is rarely linear. Celebrate consistency, not perfection.

The Science of Movement and Blood Sugar

When you move, your muscles need energy. They draw glucose from your bloodstream, lowering blood sugar levels both during and after exercise. Regular activity also helps your body use insulin more efficiently, making it a key player in reversing type 2 diabetes.

Research has shown that even **short post-meal walks** can significantly blunt blood sugar spikes. In Japan, the practice of "Sansan Taiso"—a brisk walk after meals—is a tradition that aligns beautifully with modern diabetes science.

```
- Just 30 minutes of moderate exercise a day can reduce insulin resistance and
improve blood sugar control.
- Resistance training increases muscle mass, which burns more glucose—even at
rest.
```

Building an exercise routine isn't about drastic changes or athletic feats—it's about creating a sustainable, enjoyable pattern of movement that fits your life. Whether you start with gentle stretching, neighborhood walks, or group classes, every step brings you closer to better health and greater confidence in managing your diabetes. As you grow stronger, you'll discover that movement is not just medicine—it's empowerment.

In the next section, we'll explore how to fine-tune your routine to maximize blood sugar control, and how to listen to your body's cues to prevent burnout or injury. Your journey to lasting health continues, one mindful movement at a time.

8.4 Overcoming Barriers to Activity

For many, the idea of regular exercise conjures images of crowded gyms, intimidating routines, or unending time commitments. It's natural to feel overwhelmed, especially if you're new to physical activity or managing other health challenges alongside type 2 diabetes. Yet, the path to reversing diabetes is as much about overcoming mental and practical barriers as it is about finding the right workout. Let's explore how real people have surmounted these common obstacles—and how you can, too.

Understanding Common Hurdles

Barriers to physical activity are rarely just about motivation. They often stem from a mix of personal, social, and environmental factors:

- **Time constraints** due to work, family, or other obligations.
- **Physical limitations** such as joint pain, fatigue, or mobility issues.
- **Emotional hurdles** like fear of failure, embarrassment, or lack of confidence.
- **Access issues**—living in areas without safe spaces or resources for exercise.
- **Cultural expectations** that may prioritize other duties over self-care.

Recognizing these barriers is the first step toward overcoming them. Let's look at some strategies and inspiring examples.

Key Takeaway: Small, consistent steps can lead to big changes—both personally and within your community.

Practical Strategies for Every Lifestyle

No matter your circumstances, you can tailor activity to fit your needs, abilities, and resources.

- **Break it up:** Short bouts of movement (5-10 minutes) throughout the day are as effective as longer sessions.
- **Make it social:** Involve friends, family, or coworkers for accountability and fun.
- **Adapt to your environment:** Use what's available—stairs, parks, living rooms, or even a sturdy chair.
- **Choose what you enjoy:** Dancing, gardening, swimming, or gentle yoga all count.
- **Celebrate progress:** Track small victories, like improved stamina or lower blood sugar, to stay motivated.

Historical Perspective: Movement as Medicine

Throughout history, physical activity has been woven into daily life. In traditional Japanese culture, older adults practice *rajio taiso*—a morning group calisthenics routine broadcast nationally since the 1920s. The program's enduring popularity stems from its simplicity, accessibility, and communal spirit, proving that even modest, regular movement can yield profound health benefits.

This approach contrasts with the modern, often sedentary lifestyle, but it highlights a crucial truth: sustainable activity doesn't require high-tech equipment or rigorous programs. Instead, it thrives on inclusivity, routine, and the support of others.

Navigating Physical and Emotional Obstacles

If you face pain or mobility challenges, focus on gentle movements:

- **Chair exercises** or water aerobics reduce joint stress.
- **Stretching routines** boost flexibility and circulation.
- **Mind-body practices** like tai chi improve balance and reduce anxiety.

When emotional hurdles arise—be it fear, discouragement, or self-doubt—remember that setbacks are part of every journey. Connecting with support groups or a healthcare provider can provide encouragement and guidance.

Bridging Cultural and Social Gaps

In some cultures, household responsibilities or caregiving take precedence over self-care. Harness these roles as opportunities for movement—playing with children, walking to the market, or tending a garden all contribute to your activity goals.

Building Lasting Habits

Consistency, not perfection, is the goal. Use these steps to integrate activity into your life:

- Identify one barrier you're facing.
- Choose a realistic, enjoyable activity.
- Set a small, attainable goal for the week.
- Enlist support from family or friends.
- Reflect on your progress and adjust as needed.

The journey to reversing type 2 diabetes is about persistence and self-compassion as much as movement itself.

```
Fact: Just 30 minutes of moderate activity a day can reduce insulin resistance
and improve blood sugar control—even if broken into three 10-minute sessions.
```

Overcoming barriers to activity is a deeply personal process shaped by your environment, culture, and mindset. By celebrating small wins, seeking support, and adapting routines to your life, you'll transform movement from a chore into a powerful tool for health. In our next section, we'll explore how to craft a sustainable, personalized exercise plan—one that honors where you are while guiding you toward lasting wellness.

8.5 Global Approaches to Active Living

Across the globe, the rhythm of daily life has shaped how people move—and, by extension, how they manage their health. When we look beyond our own borders, we find a wealth of insight into the connection between physical activity and metabolic well-being. These global approaches offer both inspiration and practical strategies for reversing type 2 diabetes, reminding us that movement is not just a prescription but a way of life.

Lessons from the Blue Zones

Some of the most compelling evidence about the benefits of active living comes from the so-called **Blue Zones**—regions where people live significantly longer, healthier lives. In places like Okinawa, Japan, and Sardinia, Italy, residents rarely set aside time for formal exercise. Instead, their daily routines are infused with natural movement: gardening, walking to market, tending livestock, or cycling to visit friends.

A case in point is Okinawa, where elders practice **"ikigai,"** a Japanese concept meaning "reason for being." Their days are filled with purposeful activities: working in vegetable gardens, preparing traditional meals, and engaging in community dances. Studies have shown that these gentle, consistent movements help regulate blood sugar and improve insulin sensitivity, factors deeply relevant for type 2 diabetes reversal.

Traditional Activity in Africa and South Asia

In rural Kenya, community members often walk several miles daily—not as exercise, but as necessity. Similarly, in parts of South Asia, traditional forms of movement like **yoga** and **folk dancing** are embedded in cultural rituals and celebrations. These activities, while pleasurable and socially engaging, also contribute to improved cardiovascular health and glucose regulation.

One notable example is **Surya Namaskar** (Sun Salutation), a sequence of yoga poses performed at dawn in India. This ancient practice not only enhances flexibility and strength but has been shown in modern studies to lower fasting blood sugar and improve insulin action—key targets in diabetes management.

The Science Behind Culturally Rooted Movement

What unites these diverse global approaches is a seamless integration of movement into daily existence. Research confirms that frequent, low-to-moderate intensity activity can be even more effective for blood sugar control than sporadic bouts of vigorous exercise. The secret lies in **consistency**—the kind of steady, varied activity that keeps muscles engaged and metabolism humming throughout the day.

> **Incidental activity** (movement that occurs as a byproduct of daily living) can add up to impressive totals, sometimes surpassing 10,000 steps per day.
>
> **Social engagement** is a powerful motivator. Activities done in groups—whether tai chi in a Chinese park or salsa dancing in Colombia—are more likely to be sustained over time.

Adapting Global Wisdom to Your Life

You don't need to move to Okinawa or Amsterdam to benefit from these lessons. The principles of active living can be adapted to any setting:

- Make walking a priority: Choose stairs over elevators, park farther from entrances, or explore your neighborhood on foot.
- Embrace purposeful tasks: Gardening, cleaning, or home repairs all count toward daily movement goals.
- Seek social movement: Join a walking group, dance class, or community sports league.
- Use tradition as inspiration: Try yoga, tai chi, or folk dancing—activities proven to support metabolic health.

Embracing Diversity in Active Living

Physical activity isn't "one size fits all." Your culture, interests, and environment shape the activities that feel natural and sustainable. By drawing inspiration from global traditions, you can discover forms of movement that are joyful, meaningful, and—most importantly—effective in reversing type 2 diabetes.

```
Fact: Consistent, moderate daily movement—such as brisk walking or cycling—can
lower blood sugar and reduce the need for diabetes medication, regardless of
age or fitness level.
```

8.6 Staying Safe While Exercising

Engaging in regular physical activity is a powerful tool for reversing type 2 diabetes, but safety must always come first. For people living with diabetes, the landscape of exercise includes unique challenges—blood sugar fluctuations, medication interactions, and underlying health conditions. With thoughtful preparation and a few mindful strategies, you can confidently turn movement into medicine, harnessing its benefits without unnecessary risk.

Know Your Body's Signals

Before lacing up your sneakers, it's essential to understand how your body communicates during physical exertion. Type 2 diabetes can alter the way you experience fatigue, thirst, or even pain. Pay close attention to:

- **Hypoglycemia symptoms:** Shakiness, sweating, sudden hunger, confusion, or rapid heartbeat, especially if you take insulin or certain oral medications.
- **Hyperglycemia symptoms:** Excessive thirst, frequent urination, blurred vision, or headache.
- **Unusual fatigue or dizziness:** These could signal dehydration, low blood sugar, or other issues that require attention.

Learning to recognize and respond to these signals can prevent minor discomforts from becoming emergencies.

Preparing for Safe Exercise

Preparation is half the battle in safe, effective exercise. Here's a simple checklist to guide your pre-workout routine:

Check Your Blood Sugar:

- If you're on medications that lower blood glucose, test before and after activity.
- For most, safe pre-exercise levels are 100–250 mg/dL. Below 100 mg/dL? Eat a small snack first. Above 250 mg/dL, check for ketones and consult your healthcare provider.

Wear Appropriate Gear:

- Choose well-fitting shoes to prevent blisters or foot injuries, especially important if you have neuropathy.
- Dress for the weather and environment to avoid overheating or chills.

Stay Hydrated:

- Drink water before, during, and after exercise. Dehydration can raise blood sugar and increase risk of complications.

Carry Identification:

- Wear a medical ID bracelet or carry a card noting your diabetes, medications, and emergency contacts.

Pack a Snack:

- Bring a quick-acting carbohydrate source—glucose tablets, juice, or hard candy—in case of hypoglycemia.

Adapting Activity for Special Considerations

Not all exercise is created equal, and certain conditions require additional modifications:

Neuropathy: Choose low-impact activities like swimming or cycling to protect your feet and joints.

Heart Disease: Always warm up and cool down; avoid extreme exertion and consult your physician before starting new routines.

Retinopathy: Avoid high-impact or jarring activities that increase blood pressure, like heavy lifting, which could aggravate eye issues.

If you are new to exercise or have additional health concerns, work with a healthcare provider or certified exercise professional. Many community centers and diabetes clinics offer tailored programs.

Timeline: Responding to Low Blood Sugar During Exercise

- **Notice Symptoms:** Shakiness, sweating, dizziness, or weakness.
- **Stop Activity:** Sit down in a safe place.
- **Check Blood Sugar:** If possible, use a glucose meter.
- **Treat Hypoglycemia:** Consume 15 grams of fast-acting carbohydrate (such as 4 ounces of juice or glucose tablets).
- **Wait 15 Minutes:** Recheck blood sugar. If still low, repeat treatment.
- **Resume Activity Cautiously:** Only if you feel well and blood sugar has normalized.

Community Wisdom: Global Perspectives

In India, yoga has long been integrated into diabetes care, with practitioners emphasizing mindful movement and gentle stretching. A study in Chennai found that regular yoga, when practiced with attention to hydration and blood sugar monitoring, improved glycemic control without increasing the risk of hypoglycemia. Meanwhile, in Sweden's urban centers, group walking clubs for people with diabetes offer not just physical activity, but peer support and shared safety tips—like checking in before and after each walk and carrying snacks in the group leader's backpack.

Key Safety Reminders

- Always consult your healthcare provider before starting or changing your exercise routine.
- If you experience chest pain, severe shortness of breath, or fainting, seek medical attention immediately.
- Don't let fear prevent you from moving—start slow, stay prepared, and build confidence with each step.

Fact: Exercise can lower blood sugar for up to 24 hours after activity, so monitoring levels post-workout is just as important as checking before.

Staying safe while exercising empowers you to fully reap the benefits of movement—improved blood sugar control, better mood, and greater energy—without putting your health at risk. Preparation, awareness, and learning from the experiences of others are your best allies on this journey. Next, we'll tackle the common barriers to consistent movement and strategies to sustain your motivation, helping you transform safe exercise into an enduring habit and a cornerstone of lasting health.

9 : Beyond Diet and Exercise – Stress, Sleep, and Emotional Health

9.1 The Impact of Stress on Blood Sugar

Stress is an inescapable reality of modern life. Whether it comes from work deadlines, family responsibilities, financial worries, or navigating health challenges, stress affects everyone in some way. But for those managing type 2 diabetes, stress is not merely an emotional state—it is a powerful physiological force that can directly impact blood sugar control. To understand this connection, we must explore what stress is, how the body responds to it, and why it matters so profoundly for diabetes management.

When your body perceives a threat—whether real or imagined—it triggers the **fight-or-flight response**. This ancient biological mechanism, designed to help our ancestors survive physical dangers, involves the rapid release of hormones such as **cortisol** and **adrenaline**. These hormones prompt the liver to release glucose (sugar) into the bloodstream, providing immediate energy for action. While this response was once essential for fleeing predators, today's stressors are more likely to be psychological, yet the body reacts the same way.

Stress and Blood Sugar: The Scientific Connection

For people with type 2 diabetes, the stress response can be particularly problematic. Elevated stress hormones cause:

Stress Response in Type 2 Diabetes

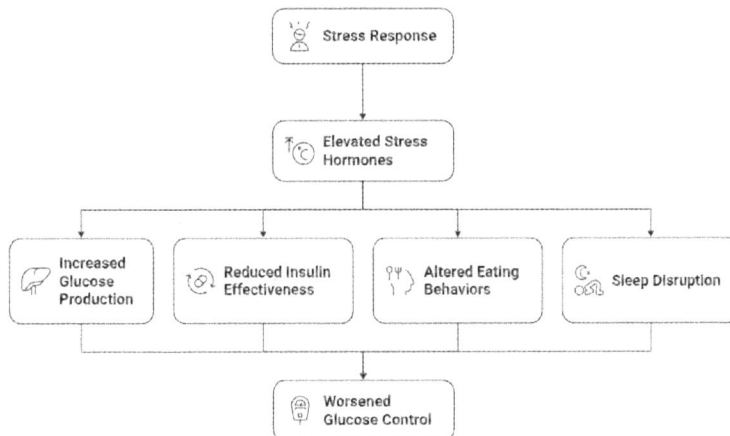

- Increased glucose production by the liver
- Reduced effectiveness of insulin (insulin resistance)

- Altered eating behaviors, often leading to unhealthy food choices
- Sleep disruption, which further worsens glucose control

When these factors combine, blood sugar levels can spike unpredictably, even if your diet and exercise routines remain stable. This can create a frustrating cycle: high blood sugar increases stress, and stress, in turn, raises blood sugar.

The Biological Chain Reaction

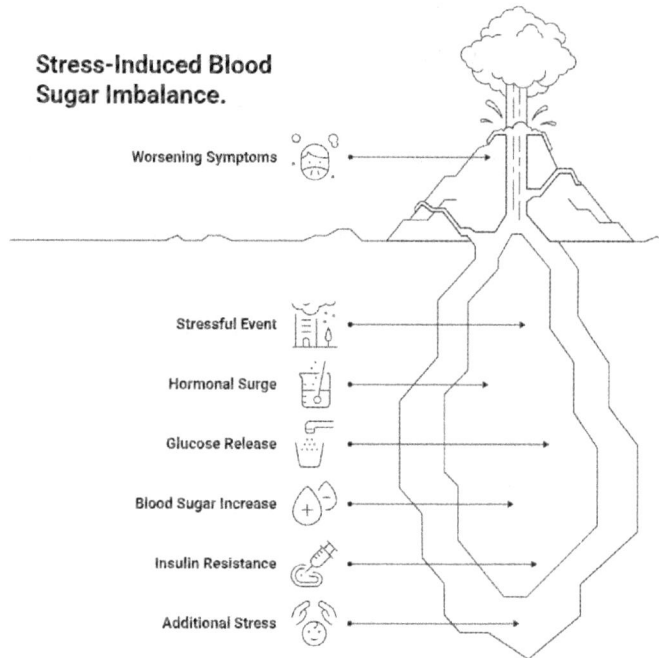

Stress-Induced Blood Sugar Imbalance.

- **Stressful Event** (work conflict, financial worry)
- **Hormonal Surge** (cortisol, adrenaline)
- **Liver Releases Glucose**
- **Increased Blood Sugar Levels**
- **Insulin Resistance Intensifies**
- **Symptoms Worsen** (fatigue, frequent urination, irritability)
- **Additional Stress**

This sequence highlights why managing stress is not an optional extra, but a core component of effective diabetes care.

Real-World Stories: The Human Face of Stress

Consider **Maria**, a teacher in Mexico City, who had managed her type 2 diabetes well for years through careful diet and regular exercise. When a sudden family emergency forced her to care for her aging parents and take on extra work, her stress levels soared. Despite sticking to her meal plan, she noticed her blood sugar readings climbing. It wasn't until she started practicing daily mindfulness meditation and sought support from her community that her glucose levels began to stabilize again.

In another example, **David**, a retiree in London, experienced chronic stress after the unexpected loss of a close friend. His grief, coupled with disrupted sleep and poor appetite, led to erratic blood sugar swings. Through grief counseling and gentle yoga, David learned to process his emotions and gradually regained control of his diabetes.

These stories are not unique. Across cultures and continents, the interplay between emotional health and metabolic health is becoming increasingly recognized by healthcare professionals and patients alike.

Cultural Perspectives on Stress and Diabetes

Different cultures respond to stress in their own ways, influencing how people with diabetes experience and manage their condition.

In **Japan**, the concept of **"karoshi"** (death by overwork) highlights the health dangers of chronic occupational stress. Japanese diabetes clinics often incorporate group relaxation therapies, such as forest bathing ("shinrin-yoku"), into their care plans.

Among **Indigenous Australian** communities, diabetes management programs include storytelling and connection to land as tools for emotional healing, recognizing that cultural loss and historical trauma contribute to stress and chronic disease.

These diverse approaches underscore the importance of addressing stress in a way that honors individual backgrounds and community values.

Recognizing Stress: Symptoms and Self-Awareness

Identifying stress is the first step toward managing it. Common signs include:

- Persistent worry or anxiety
- Difficulty sleeping or frequent waking
- Changes in appetite or food cravings
- Irritability or mood swings
- Physical symptoms like headaches, muscle tension, or stomach upset

For those with type 2 diabetes, it is especially important to monitor how stress affects blood sugar readings. Keeping a **stress diary**—noting stressful events, emotional responses, and glucose levels—can reveal patterns and help guide interventions.

Practical Strategies: Managing Stress for Blood Sugar Health

Successfully reducing stress involves both immediate relief and long-term changes. Here are evidence-based strategies:

Steps to Reduce Stress for Blood Sugar Health

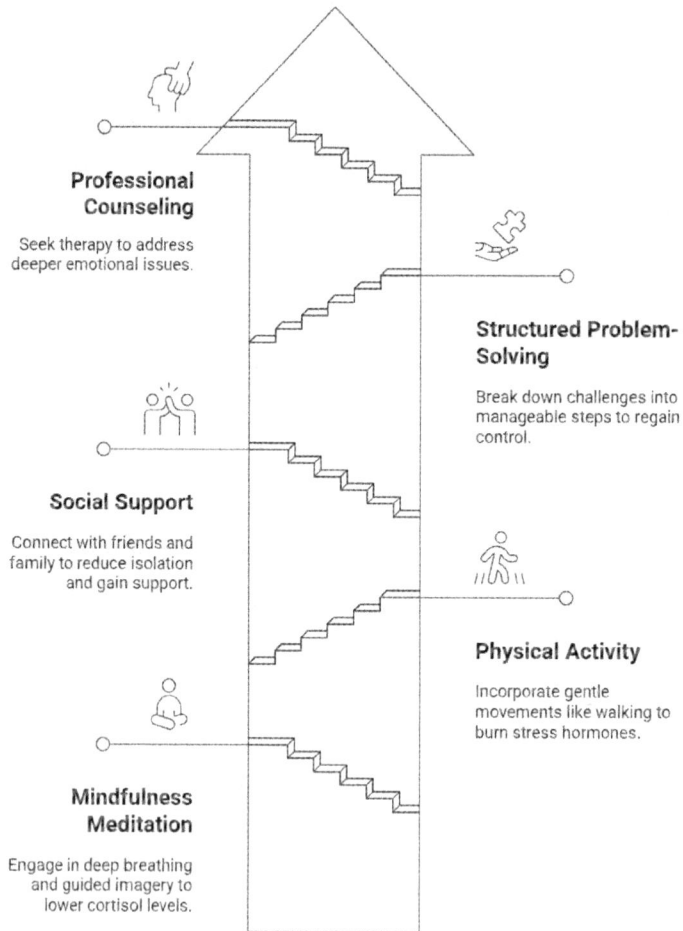

Professional Counseling

Seek therapy to address deeper emotional issues.

Structured Problem-Solving

Break down challenges into manageable steps to regain control.

Social Support

Connect with friends and family to reduce isolation and gain support.

Physical Activity

Incorporate gentle movements like walking to burn stress hormones.

Mindfulness Meditation

Engage in deep breathing and guided imagery to lower cortisol levels.

- **Mindfulness Meditation:** Techniques such as deep breathing, body scans, or guided imagery can reduce cortisol levels and improve glucose control.
- **Physical Activity:** Even gentle movement, like walking or stretching, helps burn off stress hormones and supports insulin sensitivity.

- **Social Support:** Connecting with friends, family, or support groups reduces isolation and provides practical help during difficult times.
- **Structured Problem-Solving:** Breaking down overwhelming challenges into smaller, manageable steps restores a sense of control.
- **Professional Counseling:** Therapists or counselors can help address deeper issues such as grief, anxiety, or trauma.

Adopting one or more of these strategies can transform the way you handle stress and positively influence your diabetes management.

```
- Chronic stress can raise blood sugar levels—even if you haven't changed your
diet or exercise habits.
- Stress management is as crucial as medication, diet, and exercise in
reversing type 2 diabetes.
```

Stress is invisible but powerful, weaving its way into every aspect of diabetes management. By recognizing the impact of stress on blood sugar and taking proactive steps to address it, you reclaim a vital part of your health journey. As we continue, the next section will explore the equally important roles of sleep and emotional well-being, further equipping you with the tools for lasting health and resilience on your path to reversing type 2 diabetes.

9.2 Sleep and Diabetes

Sleep is often the unsung hero of health, quietly working behind the scenes to restore, repair, and regulate the body. For those living with type 2 diabetes—or striving to reverse it—getting quality sleep is not simply a luxury, but a crucial component of metabolic control. As we have learned, managing stress and emotional well-being can have a profound impact on blood sugar levels. Yet, without adequate sleep, even the best dietary and exercise efforts might fall short of their full potential.

The Science Connecting Sleep and Blood Sugar

The relationship between sleep and diabetes is both intimate and intricate. During restful sleep, the body undergoes essential hormonal balancing: insulin sensitivity improves, stress hormone levels like cortisol decrease, and the body's energy stores are replenished. When sleep is disrupted—through insomnia, sleep apnea, or simply not enough hours in bed—these processes are thrown off balance.

- **Insulin Resistance:** Chronic sleep deprivation has been shown to increase insulin resistance, making it harder for your body to process glucose efficiently.

- **Appetite Hormones:** Lack of sleep alters levels of ghrelin and leptin, hormones that regulate hunger and satiety, often leading to increased appetite and cravings for high-sugar, high-fat foods.
- **Inflammation:** Poor sleep increases inflammation throughout the body, further impairing metabolic health and promoting the progression of diabetes.

A landmark study conducted at the University of Chicago in the early 2000s found that even a single week of restricted sleep caused otherwise healthy adults to exhibit glucose tolerance levels similar to those seen in prediabetes. These findings underscore just how quickly poor sleep can undermine metabolic health.

Common Sleep Disruptors in Diabetes

People with type 2 diabetes often face unique challenges that can interfere with restful sleep. Understanding these obstacles is a critical step toward improvement.

- **Nocturia:** High blood sugar can cause frequent urination at night, interrupting sleep cycles.
- **Restless Legs Syndrome:** Diabetes-related nerve damage (neuropathy) can cause uncomfortable sensations in the legs, making it hard to fall or stay asleep.
- **Obstructive Sleep Apnea:** This condition, more common in those with excess weight and diabetes, causes repeated pauses in breathing during sleep, leading to frequent awakenings and poor sleep quality.

Consider the story of **José**, a 54-year-old schoolteacher from Brazil. After years of struggling with fatigue and high morning blood sugar, he was diagnosed with obstructive sleep apnea. With the help of a sleep specialist and the use of a CPAP machine, José's sleep quality improved dramatically—and so did his blood sugar control. His experience is a powerful reminder that sometimes, addressing sleep issues unlocks the door to better diabetes management.

Strategies for Restoring Restful Sleep

Improving sleep is both an art and a science. For many, small lifestyle adjustments can yield big benefits:

Unveiling Strategies for Restful Sleep

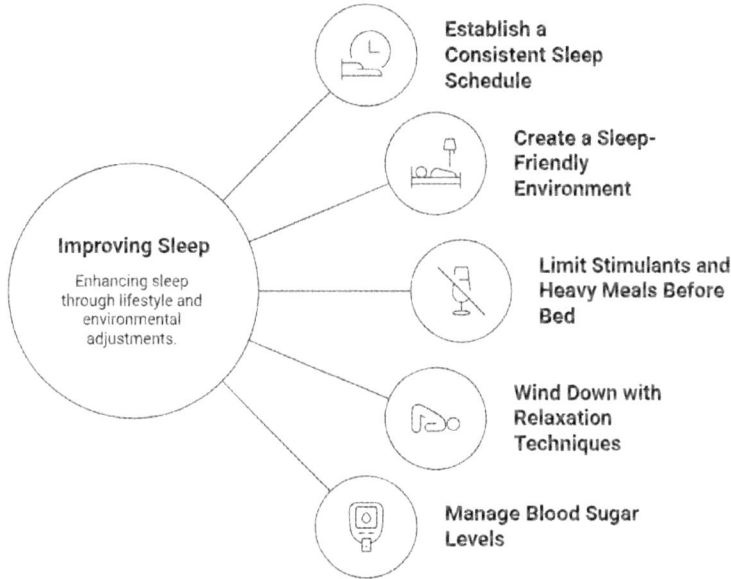

- **Establish a Consistent Sleep Schedule**

  - Go to bed and wake up at the same time every day, even on weekends.
  - This helps regulate your body's internal clock and improves sleep quality.

- **Create a Sleep-Friendly Environment**

  - Keep your bedroom dark, cool, and quiet.
  - Remove electronic devices that emit light or noise.

- **Limit Stimulants and Heavy Meals Before Bed**

  - Avoid caffeine and large, high-sugar meals in the evening.
  - Alcohol can also disrupt sleep patterns, even if it makes you drowsy initially.

- **Wind Down with Relaxation Techniques**

  - Gentle yoga, meditation, or deep breathing exercises before bed can signal to your body that it's time to sleep.
  - Reading or listening to calming music may also help.

- **Manage Blood Sugar Levels**

- Monitor your nighttime blood sugar and discuss any concerns with your healthcare provider.
- Having stable blood sugar at night reduces nighttime awakenings due to hypoglycemia or hyperglycemia.

Global Perspectives: Sleep and Diabetes Around the World

Sleep challenges in diabetes are not limited by geography. In India, for example, rapid urbanization and longer work hours have led to a surge in both type 2 diabetes and sleep disorders. A 2018 study in Mumbai found that nearly 40% of adults with type 2 diabetes reported poor sleep quality—a statistic mirrored in many urban centers worldwide. Cultural practices, such as late-night meals or irregular work shifts, can further complicate sleep hygiene.

In Japan, the concept of **inemuri**—napping in public places—is socially accepted and even encouraged as a sign of diligence. While short daytime naps can be restorative, chronic lack of nighttime sleep remains a problem, especially among the working population, and has been linked to higher rates of metabolic diseases, including type 2 diabetes. These examples remind us that while the context may differ, the fundamental need for quality sleep is universal.

When to Seek Professional Help

Sometimes, despite best efforts, sleep problems persist. It's important to recognize when to seek medical advice:

Persistent insomnia (difficulty falling or staying asleep for more than a month)
Loud snoring, choking, or gasping during sleep (possible sleep apnea)
Unexplained daytime sleepiness or fatigue

A healthcare provider may recommend a sleep study or further evaluation. Addressing underlying sleep disorders not only improves quality of life but can be a pivotal step toward reversing type 2 diabetes.

```
- Chronic sleep deprivation can worsen insulin resistance and blood sugar
control, undermining efforts to reverse type 2 diabetes.
- Addressing sleep issues—such as sleep apnea or insomnia—can significantly
improve diabetes management and overall well-being.
```

Sleep is a foundation of health, influencing everything from hormonal balance to daily energy levels. For those on the journey to reverse type 2 diabetes, prioritizing restful sleep is not optional—it's essential. By creating healthy sleep habits and seeking help for persistent problems, you empower your body to heal and thrive.

As we move forward, the next section will delve into the often-overlooked realm of emotional well-being, exploring how mind and mood can support—or sabotage—your progress. Understanding this final piece of the puzzle will help you achieve not just better numbers, but a more vibrant, resilient life.

9.3 Emotional Health and Diabetes

Our emotional landscape is an often-overlooked factor in the journey to reverse type 2 diabetes, yet it is as influential as dietary choices, exercise, and sleep. The intricate interplay between the mind and body becomes especially apparent when we consider how stress, anxiety, and mood disturbances can affect blood sugar levels and overall health outcomes. Tackling emotional health isn't just about seeking happiness—it's about creating a stable, supportive environment for lasting physiological change.

The Science Behind Emotions and Blood Sugar

Emotions are not just fleeting feelings; they trigger real, measurable changes in the body. When you feel threatened or overwhelmed, your body initiates the **stress response**—a cascade of hormonal changes designed for survival. Key among these hormones is **cortisol**, which signals your liver to release glucose into the bloodstream, providing energy for a "fight or flight" response. While this mechanism helped our ancestors evade predators, for modern individuals with type 2 diabetes, repeated activation can lead to persistent high blood sugar.

- **Chronic Stress:** Prolonged emotional stress can lead to sustained high cortisol levels, making it more difficult to manage blood glucose, even with a healthy diet and regular exercise.
- **Anxiety and Depression:** Studies have shown that people with diabetes are twice as likely to experience depression, which can create a vicious cycle—depression leads to neglect of self-care, making diabetes management harder, which in turn fuels more emotional distress.

Emotional Health Strategies for Diabetes Management

Emotional well-being can be cultivated with intentional strategies that fit diverse lifestyles, cultures, and personal histories. Some approaches are rooted in modern psychology, while others draw upon longstanding traditions from around the world.

- **Mindfulness and Meditation:** Practices like mindfulness meditation have been shown in numerous studies to decrease stress, lower anxiety, and even improve glycemic control. Mindful eating, in particular, can help individuals recognize hunger cues and avoid emotional eating—a common challenge in diabetes management.

- **Cognitive Behavioral Therapy (CBT):** CBT is a structured approach to identifying and changing negative thought patterns. For people with diabetes, CBT can reduce depression and improve self-care behaviors.
- **Social Connection:** Isolation can worsen both mood and blood sugar. Building a network—whether through family, friends, community groups, or online forums—provides emotional support and practical tips for daily management.
- **Cultural Healing Practices:** In many cultures, emotional healing is intertwined with spirituality, art, or communal rituals. For instance, Native American talking circles or West African drumming groups offer safe spaces for emotional expression, connection, and healing.

Timeline: The Emotional Health–Diabetes Connection

Diagnosis: Feelings of fear, confusion, or denial are common. Emotional support at this stage can set the tone for proactive management.

Early Management: Motivation is high, but frustration may arise with setbacks. Peer support or counseling can help maintain positive momentum.

Long-term Maintenance: Emotional fatigue or "diabetes burnout" can emerge. Renewed focus on stress reduction, self-compassion, and social connection is crucial for sustaining progress.

Historical Perspective: Banting's Emotional Resilience

The story of **Sir Frederick Banting**, co-discoverer of insulin, is a testament to the power of emotional resilience. Banting faced repeated setbacks, skepticism, and financial strain during his research. Yet, his determination and ability to manage stress not only led to a breakthrough but also changed millions of lives. His journey reminds us that emotional strength is not just a personal asset—it can drive transformative change for others as well.

Global Perspective: Emotional Health in Different Cultures

Approaches to emotional health and diabetes care vary worldwide:

- In **Japan**, the practice of **shinrin-yoku** (forest bathing) is widely embraced to reduce stress and restore emotional balance, with measurable benefits for blood pressure and glucose control.
- In **Mexico**, traditional family meals and community gatherings provide a sense of belonging and emotional nourishment, helping individuals manage the psychological demands of living with a chronic illness.

- In **Sweden**, open conversations about mental health are encouraged in healthcare settings, reducing stigma and enabling patients to access counseling as part of diabetes care.

These examples highlight that emotional well-being is not a luxury—it is a universal need, and its fulfillment can look different across cultures.

Practical Tips for Building Emotional Resilience

- **Practice gratitude daily:** Even noting three things you're thankful for can shift your mindset.
- **Schedule regular relaxation:** Whether through yoga, music, or quiet reflection, prioritize downtime.
- **Seek professional help if needed:** Don't hesitate to speak with a counselor or psychologist; many have experience supporting people with chronic health conditions.
- **Set realistic goals:** Celebrate small victories in your diabetes journey, and be gentle with yourself during setbacks.

How to build emotional resilience?

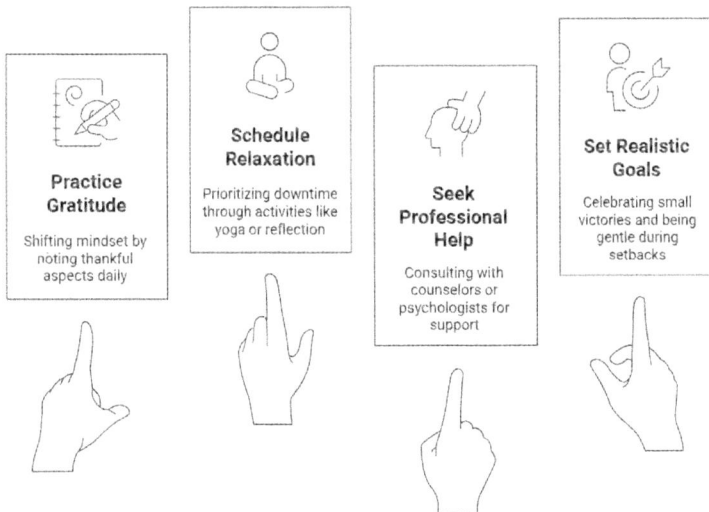

Practice Gratitude
Shifting mindset by noting thankful aspects daily

Schedule Relaxation
Prioritizing downtime through activities like yoga or reflection

Seek Professional Help
Consulting with counselors or psychologists for support

Set Realistic Goals
Celebrating small victories and being gentle during setbacks

Important: Chronic stress and emotional distress can significantly raise blood sugar levels, undermining even the best diet and exercise plans. Prioritizing emotional well-being is essential for sustained diabetes reversal.

In summary, emotional health is not simply an adjunct to physical well-being— it is a fundamental pillar in your path to reversing type 2 diabetes. By recognizing and nurturing your emotional needs, you are not only optimizing your blood sugar control but also enriching your life with resilience, connection, and hope.

As we turn the page to our next chapter, we will explore how sustainable lifestyle routines—built on the foundation of physical, emotional, and social well-being—can empower you to maintain your progress long after the initial excitement fades. The path to lasting health is not a sprint, but a journey, and every aspect of your life plays a role in your success.

9.4 Integrative Approaches

In the journey to reverse type 2 diabetes, diet and exercise are essential pillars, but they are not the only ones holding up the structure of lasting health. As we've seen, sustaining progress requires a holistic perspective—one that acknowledges the intricate interplay between mind, body, and spirit. Integrative approaches bridge these elements, drawing on diverse tools and traditions to support not just physical change, but total well-being. By focusing on stress management, restorative sleep, and emotional resilience, we can unlock deeper, more enduring transformation.

Understanding the Mind-Body Connection

For centuries, healers across the world have recognized the profound connection between emotional health and physical disease. Today, scientific research confirms what ancient wisdom suggested: chronic stress, poor sleep, and emotional turmoil can all drive blood sugar dysregulation and inflammation, undermining your best efforts at dietary or fitness change.

- **Chronic stress** triggers the release of cortisol and other hormones that raise blood glucose.
- **Sleep deprivation** impairs insulin sensitivity, making it harder for your body to regulate sugar.
- **Emotional distress** can lead to unhealthy eating patterns and decreased motivation for self-care.

The mind and body are not separate in the context of diabetes—they are partners in the healing process.

Stress Reduction: Practices and Perspectives

Modern life is filled with stressors, from work deadlines to family responsibilities, financial worries to social pressures. How you respond to these challenges can dramatically affect your health outcomes.

Mindfulness meditation is one of the most researched and accessible tools for stress management. Developed from ancient Buddhist traditions, mindfulness invites you to pay attention to the present moment without judgment. In a landmark study at the University of Massachusetts, Dr. Jon Kabat-Zinn's Mindfulness-Based Stress Reduction (MBSR) program was shown to lower blood sugar levels and improve overall well-being in people with type 2 diabetes.

Yoga is another integrative practice, blending physical movement with breath work and mental focus. In India, where yoga originated, researchers have found that regular practice leads to reduced fasting glucose and improved insulin sensitivity. Even gentle yoga, practiced for 15-30 minutes daily, can foster calm and help regulate stress hormones.

Breathwork techniques, such as diaphragmatic breathing or alternate nostril breathing (pranayama), offer rapid relief from acute stress. By slowing the breath and focusing attention, you can activate the parasympathetic nervous system, which counters the body's fight-or-flight response.

Sleep: The Underestimated Healer

Sleep is the body's natural time for repair and regulation—but it's often sacrificed in the name of productivity. For those with type 2 diabetes, sleep takes on special importance.

- During deep sleep, the body restores insulin sensitivity and balances hormones.
- Chronic sleep deprivation is linked to increased appetite, cravings for sugary foods, and weight gain.
- Poor sleep raises cortisol and disrupts glucose metabolism, making blood sugar harder to control.

Sleep hygiene is the term for simple, actionable habits that improve sleep quality:

- Maintain a consistent bedtime and wake time, even on weekends.
- Limit screens and bright lights at least 30 minutes before bed.
- Keep your bedroom cool, dark, and quiet.
- Avoid caffeine and large meals within several hours of sleep.

In Japan, where the concept of "inemuri" (napping in public) is culturally accepted, researchers have found that short daytime naps can reduce stress and improve metabolic health—provided they don't interfere with nighttime sleep.

Emotional Resilience: Building Inner Strength

Managing a chronic condition like type 2 diabetes can be emotionally taxing. Feelings of frustration, guilt, or hopelessness are common, but they don't have to define your journey. Developing emotional resilience—the ability to bounce back from setbacks—is critical for long-term success.

Consider the story of **Maria**, a 54-year-old teacher living in Argentina. After her diagnosis, Maria struggled with self-blame and anxiety. Through participation in a local diabetes support group, she learned to reframe her experience: diabetes was not a punishment, but a challenge she could meet with curiosity and courage. By practicing gratitude journaling and reaching out for help, Maria regained control over her emotions and, with time, her blood sugar. Her story echoes findings from multiple studies: people who connect with supportive communities and cultivate positive emotions are more likely to sustain healthy habits and see improvements in their diabetes markers.

Integrative Therapies Around the World

Globally, communities have developed unique approaches to healing mind and body together:

- In **Finland**, forest bathing (spending mindful time in natural settings) is used to reduce stress and lower blood pressure—an approach now gaining popularity worldwide.
- In **China**, traditional Tai Chi combines gentle movement, breath, and focus to improve balance, reduce anxiety, and support glucose control.

These traditions remind us that healing is not just about what we eat or how we move, but how we nurture our inner landscape.

Bringing It All Together: Your Personal Toolbox

Integrative approaches are not about abandoning science or replacing medicine with mysticism. Instead, they are about expanding your toolbox—adding evidence-backed practices that complement your diet, exercise, and medication (if needed).

Choose one or two stress management techniques to practice regularly.

Prioritize sleep as a non-negotiable part of your health plan.

Seek emotional support through counseling, support groups, or trusted friends.

Explore global traditions for inspiration, adapting practices that resonate with your lifestyle and beliefs.

Remember, there is no "one-size-fits-all" solution—what matters is finding what works for you, and making those habits a regular part of your routine.

```
Chronic stress and sleep deprivation can raise blood sugar as much as a high-
carbohydrate meal—addressing them is just as crucial as diet for diabetes
reversal.
```

Integrative approaches remind us that reversing type 2 diabetes is not just about the numbers on a chart, but about creating harmony in our whole lives. By tending to stress, sleep, and emotional well-being, you lay the foundation for lasting change. As we move forward, let's explore how building a sustainable support network—and harnessing the power of community—can further empower you on your path to health.

9.5 Creating a Self-Care Plan

True transformation in reversing type 2 diabetes goes beyond tracking carbs or logging steps. It's about nurturing your whole self—body, mind, and spirit. While diet and exercise are powerful tools, the daily pressures of life, lack of quality sleep, and emotional turbulence can silently undermine even the most disciplined efforts. This is where the concept of **self-care** becomes essential. Self-care is not an indulgence; it is a deliberate commitment to actions and routines that protect and enhance your well-being, especially as you strive to regain control over your health.

Across cultures and histories, people have recognized the healing power of self-care. In traditional Japanese culture, the practice of **shinrin-yoku**, or "forest bathing," emphasizes the restorative effects of spending time in nature—a form of self-care that reduces stress and supports overall health. Meanwhile, in Scandinavian countries, the concept of **hygge** encourages simple pleasures and coziness, promoting emotional balance during long, dark winters. These diverse traditions remind us that self-care is both universal and deeply personal.

Key Elements of a Diabetes Self-Care Plan

A comprehensive self-care plan for reversing type 2 diabetes should address not only physical health but also psychological and social needs. Here are the fundamental components to consider:

- **Stress Management:** Chronic stress can raise blood sugar levels, disrupt hormones, and lead to emotional eating. Learning to identify and manage stress is crucial.
- **Quality Sleep:** Poor sleep affects insulin sensitivity and appetite-regulating hormones, making diabetes harder to control.

- **Emotional Well-being:** Mental health challenges, such as anxiety or depression, are common in people with diabetes and can undermine self-management efforts.
- **Support Systems:** Social support from family, friends, or community groups provides encouragement and accountability.
- **Routine Monitoring:** Regularly checking your blood sugar, tracking moods, and noting patterns can inform your self-care decisions.

Diabetes Self-Care Plan

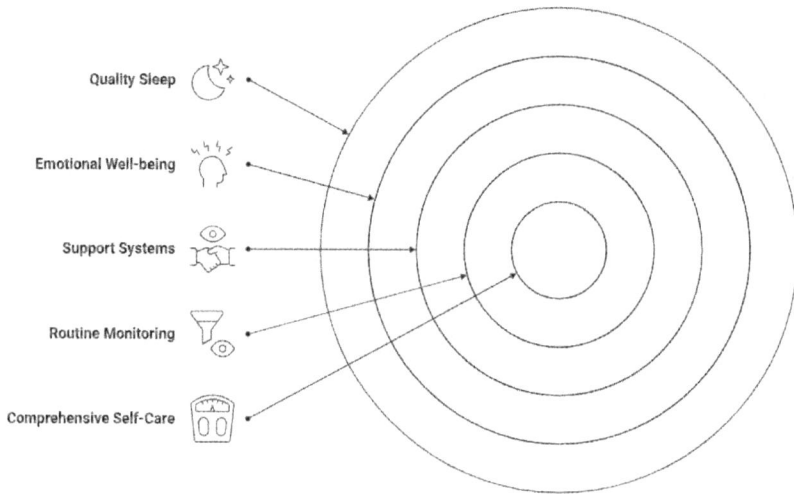

Quality Sleep

Emotional Well-being

Support Systems

Routine Monitoring

Comprehensive Self-Care

Steps to Building Your Self-Care Plan

Each person's journey is unique, but the following steps can help you develop a sustainable, personalized self-care strategy:

- **Assess Your Needs**

  - Reflect on areas where you feel most challenged: stress, sleep, emotional ups and downs, or social isolation.
  - Ask yourself: What drains my energy? What restores it? Where do I need the most support?

- **Set Realistic Goals**

  - Choose one or two small, specific goals to start. For instance, aim to meditate for five minutes a day, or set a consistent bedtime.
  - Use the SMART framework—Specific, Measurable, Achievable, Relevant, Time-bound—for clarity.

- **Select Self-Care Activities**

  - Identify activities that help you recharge. These might include:
  - Deep breathing or mindfulness exercises
  - Journaling or creative expression
  - Connecting with loved ones
  - Gentle movement, like yoga or walking in nature
  - Limiting screen time before bed

- **Create a Routine**

  - Integrate self-care into your daily schedule. For example, set a reminder for a midday stretch or evening relaxation ritual.
  - Treat these appointments with the same importance as medical check-ups.

- **Monitor and Adjust**

  - Regularly review how your plan is working. Are stress levels dropping? Is sleep improving? Adjust as needed, and celebrate progress.

Tools and Techniques for Effective Self-Care

Consider incorporating these evidence-based practices into your self-care plan:

- **Mindfulness Meditation:** Even a few minutes daily can lower stress hormones and stabilize blood sugar.
- **Sleep Hygiene:** Keep a regular sleep schedule, create a calm bedtime environment, and avoid caffeine or heavy meals late in the day.
- **Cognitive Behavioral Techniques:** Challenge negative thoughts and replace them with constructive, supportive self-talk.
- **Gratitude Journaling:** Writing down three things you're grateful for each day can shift your focus and reduce anxiety.

Cultural Considerations in Self-Care

Self-care is shaped by cultural beliefs and practices. For example, in Mediterranean regions, the tradition of a midday siesta or leisurely family meal emphasizes rest and connection—a potent antidote to modern stress. In the United States, workplace wellness programs are becoming more common, encouraging employees to take breaks for movement or relaxation.

Adapting self-care to your personal and cultural context increases the likelihood that it will become a meaningful and lasting part of your life.

Common Barriers and How to Overcome Them

Many people face obstacles when trying to prioritize self-care:

- **Time constraints:** Start small—just five minutes can make a difference.
- **Guilt or self-judgment:** Remember, self-care is not selfish; it's essential for managing diabetes.
- **Lack of support:** Reach out to friends, family, or online communities for encouragement.

By anticipating challenges and planning for them, you can create a self-care routine that fits your life.

```
- Chronic stress raises blood sugar by increasing cortisol, a hormone that
makes insulin less effective.
- Just one night of poor sleep can reduce insulin sensitivity by up to 33%,
increasing the risk of high blood sugar the next day.
```

Self-care is the bridge between knowledge and action—the daily commitment that allows you to thrive, not just survive, with type 2 diabetes. By honoring your physical, emotional, and social needs, you create a foundation for lasting health. As you continue your journey, remember that every small act of self-care is a powerful step toward reversing diabetes and reclaiming your vitality.

10 : Medication and Medical Management

10.1 Understanding Diabetes Medications

When first diagnosed with **type 2 diabetes**, many people find themselves navigating a complex world of medications with unfamiliar names and nuanced effects. While lifestyle modifications—like dietary changes, exercise, and stress management—are at the heart of reversing and controlling diabetes, medications often play a crucial role, especially in the early stages or when blood sugar levels are significantly elevated. Understanding these medications is not only empowering but essential for anyone seeking to reduce dependency on them as their health improves.

How Diabetes Medications Work

Diabetes medications are designed to lower blood glucose (sugar) levels by targeting different aspects of the body's metabolism. Broadly, these drugs either:

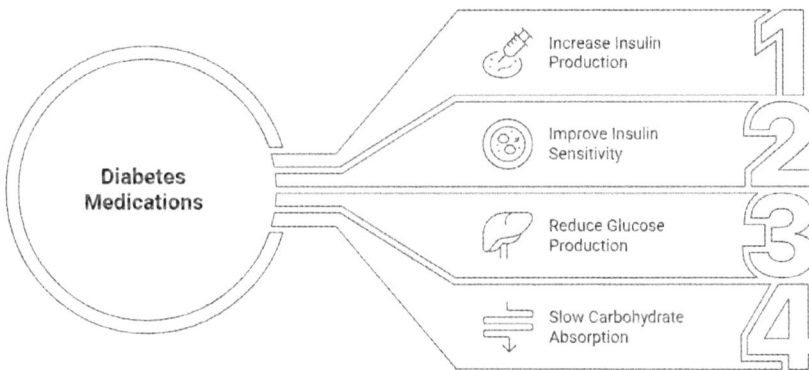

Pathways of Diabetes Medication Action

- Increase insulin production
- Improve insulin sensitivity
- Reduce glucose production by the liver
- Slow carbohydrate absorption

Let's explore the main categories:

- **Metformin:** The most commonly prescribed first-line medication worldwide, metformin works by reducing glucose production in the liver and increasing insulin sensitivity. It is typically well-tolerated and does not cause weight gain.

- **Sulfonylureas:** These stimulate the pancreas to produce more insulin. While effective, they can sometimes lead to low blood sugar (hypoglycemia) and weight gain.
- **DPP-4 Inhibitors, GLP-1 Agonists, SGLT2 Inhibitors:** Newer classes of medications that either help the body release more insulin, slow digestion, or increase glucose excretion through urine.
- **Insulin:** Some individuals may require insulin injections, especially if other medications are insufficient or if blood sugar is extremely high.

Pathways to Blood Sugar Control

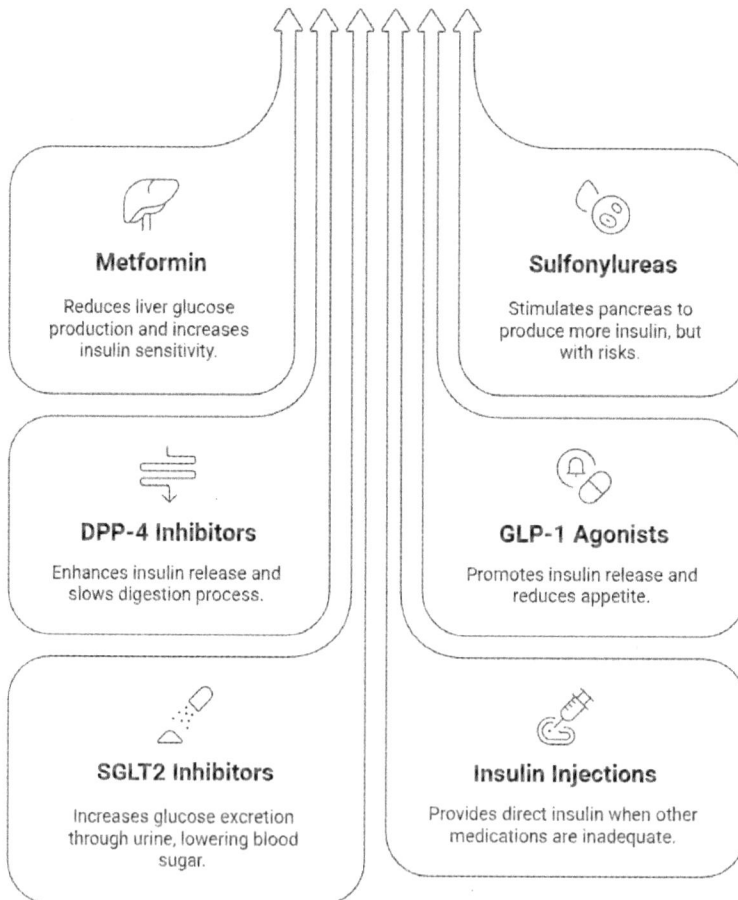

Metformin

Reduces liver glucose production and increases insulin sensitivity.

Sulfonylureas

Stimulates pancreas to produce more insulin, but with risks.

DPP-4 Inhibitors

Enhances insulin release and slows digestion process.

GLP-1 Agonists

Promotes insulin release and reduces appetite.

SGLT2 Inhibitors

Increases glucose excretion through urine, lowering blood sugar.

Insulin Injections

Provides direct insulin when other medications are inadequate.

Each medication has its own benefits and side effects, and the choice depends on individual health profiles, preferences, and often, access to healthcare resources.

A Brief History: The Evolution of Diabetes Drugs

The journey of diabetes medications is a story of scientific discovery and human resilience. In the early 20th century, before the discovery of insulin, a diagnosis of diabetes was often a death sentence. In 1921, Canadian scientists Frederick Banting and Charles Best isolated insulin, transforming diabetes care and saving countless lives—a medical breakthrough commemorated every year on World Diabetes Day.

Metformin, now a cornerstone of type 2 diabetes management, has a surprisingly long history. French lilac (Galega officinalis), a plant used in medieval Europe to treat "sweet urine," contains the compound from which metformin was eventually derived. Its use in medicine, however, did not become widespread until the mid-20th century, when it was proven to be safe and effective.

Real-World Example: Maria's Medication Journey

Consider **Maria**, a 52-year-old teacher from Mexico City. Diagnosed with type 2 diabetes five years ago, she was initially prescribed metformin and, as her blood glucose levels climbed, a sulfonylurea. Despite her best efforts, Maria felt overwhelmed by the growing list of pills and the side effects, including occasional dizziness.

After attending a diabetes education workshop in her community, Maria began making gradual but consistent changes to her diet, focusing on low glycemic index foods and regular walks in the city's parks. Within a year, her doctor noted steady improvements in her blood sugar readings. With close medical supervision, Maria was able to reduce her sulfonylurea dose and, eventually, discontinue it altogether— maintaining good control with just metformin and healthy habits.

Why Medication Reduction Matters

Reducing dependency on diabetes medications is not just about fewer pills. It reflects improved metabolic health, less risk of side effects, and—most importantly— greater autonomy and confidence in managing the condition. However, it is vital to approach medication changes carefully:

- Medications should only be reduced or discontinued under the guidance of a healthcare professional.
- Sudden changes in medication can cause dangerous fluctuations in blood sugar.

Global Perspectives on Access and Usage

Access to diabetes medications varies dramatically worldwide. In high-income countries, newer drugs are increasingly available, offering added benefits such as weight loss and cardiovascular protection. However, in many low- and middle-income regions, metformin and sulfonylureas remain the mainstay due to cost and availability. Cultural factors also shape attitudes toward medication—some communities emphasize herbal remedies or traditional healing, while others focus on biomedical approaches.

Key Takeaways for Lasting Health

- Educate yourself about your medications—know what you take, why, and what side effects to watch for.
- Remember that medication is a tool, not a life sentence: lifestyle changes can often reduce or even eliminate the need for certain drugs.
- Collaborate closely with your healthcare provider to develop a personalized plan.

```
Fact: Metformin is derived from a compound found in French lilac, a plant used
in folk medicine for centuries to treat symptoms of diabetes.
Important: Never stop or change diabetes medications without professional
medical guidance, as this can lead to life-threatening complications.
```

Understanding diabetes medications is a vital step in reclaiming your health and independence. By demystifying these tools and learning how they work, you can make informed decisions in partnership with your healthcare team. In the next section, we'll explore practical strategies for safely reducing medication dependency as blood sugar control improves, reinforcing the central message of empowerment and lasting wellness on your journey to reversing type 2 diabetes.

10.2 When Medication Is Necessary

For many individuals working toward reversing type 2 diabetes, reducing medication dependency is a meaningful goal—a testament to the power of lifestyle change and self-empowerment. However, it is crucial to recognize that medication has a vital, sometimes lifesaving, role in diabetes management. Understanding when medication is necessary ensures safety, prevents complications, and supports your body during periods when lifestyle interventions alone may not suffice.

The Essential Role of Medication

Medications, whether oral agents, injectables, or insulin, are not a sign of failure. Instead, they serve as powerful tools that help stabilize blood sugar levels, prevent dangerous spikes and drops, and protect vital organs from the damaging effects of chronic hyperglycemia. There are situations where starting or continuing medication is not only wise but absolutely essential:

- **Severely Elevated Blood Sugar**: At diagnosis, some individuals present with dangerously high blood glucose (often above 300 mg/dL or 16.7 mmol/L). Immediate medical intervention is required to prevent acute complications like diabetic ketoacidosis or hyperosmolar hyperglycemic state.

- **Symptoms of Uncontrolled Diabetes**: Persistent fatigue, frequent urination, excessive thirst, blurred vision, and unexplained weight loss are warning signs that blood sugar is not under control and medication may be needed.
- **Acute Illness or Surgery**: During times of infection, major illness, or surgery, the body's stress response can increase blood glucose, necessitating temporary or increased medication.
- **Progression of Disease**: Over time, despite best efforts, the pancreas may become less able to produce insulin, requiring pharmacological support to maintain healthy blood sugar levels.

The Safety Net: Preventing Complications

One of the most important reasons for medication is the prevention of both acute and chronic complications. Poorly controlled diabetes can lead to:

- **Cardiovascular events**, such as heart attack or stroke
- **Kidney damage** (diabetic nephropathy)
- **Vision loss** (diabetic retinopathy)
- **Nerve damage** (neuropathy)
- **Life-threatening metabolic emergencies**

By using medication judiciously, individuals can avoid these outcomes while gradually working towards health goals through diet, exercise, and stress management.

Global Perspectives: Access and Attitudes Toward Medication

Attitudes toward diabetes medication can vary across cultures. In some regions, such as Scandinavia, there is a strong emphasis on early intervention with both medication and structured education, resulting in some of the world's lowest rates of diabetes complications. In contrast, in parts of sub-Saharan Africa and South Asia, fear or stigma around medication can delay timely treatment, increasing the risk of preventable health crises.

Understanding these cultural perspectives reminds us that medication is not just a medical tool—it is also shaped by beliefs, access, and trust in the healthcare system. Advocacy for equitable, stigma-free access to medication is essential for global diabetes care.

Recognizing the Signs: When to Seek Medical Help

While self-management is empowering, it's critical to know when professional care is required. Seek immediate medical advice if you experience:

- Persistent blood sugar readings above 250 mg/dL (13.9 mmol/L)
- Symptoms of dehydration, confusion, or difficulty breathing
- Infections that do not heal, or wounds with signs of infection
- Sudden vision changes or chest pain

Early intervention can prevent emergencies and set you back on the path to wellness.

Key Points to Remember

- Medication is a safety net, not a setback. It protects your body while you pursue sustainable lifestyle changes.
- Temporary use of medication can allow you to regain control and prevent irreversible complications.
- Open communication with your healthcare provider is essential—never stop or change medications without professional guidance.

Important: Medication may be necessary during periods of high stress, illness, or when lifestyle changes alone are insufficient. Always consult your healthcare provider before making changes to your diabetes regimen.

Recognizing when medication is necessary is a cornerstone of responsible diabetes management. By embracing medications as allies—rather than adversaries—you safeguard your health while steadily working toward greater independence. As we move forward, the next section will explore how to collaborate effectively with your healthcare team, ensuring that every step of your journey is supported by expertise, compassion, and partnership.

10.3 Reducing Medication with Lifestyle Change

For many people living with type 2 diabetes, the idea of reducing or eventually eliminating diabetes medication feels like an unattainable dream. Yet, decades of research and countless personal journeys have shown that, for some, this goal is not only possible but achievable through dedicated lifestyle changes. Central to this transformation is understanding that **medication** is not a cure, but a tool—one that can often be scaled back as the body heals and responds to healthier habits.

Lifestyle modification addresses the root causes of insulin resistance and high blood sugar, targeting the underlying metabolic dysfunction rather than simply masking its symptoms. This approach is anchored in sustained improvements to diet, physical activity, weight management, and stress reduction. Let's explore how these strategies can help reduce reliance on medication and, in some cases, even reverse type 2 diabetes.

The Science Behind Lifestyle-Driven Change

Type 2 diabetes develops when the body becomes resistant to insulin, or when the pancreas cannot produce enough insulin to keep blood glucose levels in check. Medications, including metformin, sulfonylureas, and insulin injections, help manage blood sugar but do not address the factors that cause insulin resistance.

Evidence from landmark studies, such as the **Diabetes Prevention Program (DPP)** in the United States and the **DiRECT (Diabetes Remission Clinical Trial)** in the UK, shows that:

- **Weight loss**—even a modest 5-10% reduction—can significantly improve insulin sensitivity.
- **Consistent physical activity** helps muscles use glucose more efficiently, reducing blood sugar.
- **Dietary improvements** lower the glycemic load on the body, easing the burden on the pancreas.
- **Stress management** reduces levels of cortisol, a hormone that can exacerbate insulin resistance.

A Timeline for Change: From Medication to Mastery

Every individual's journey is unique, but there are common milestones on the path to reducing diabetes medication through lifestyle change:

- **Initiation (Weeks 1-4):** Begin with small, manageable adjustments such as reducing sugary foods, adding daily walks, and increasing water intake. Early wins build momentum.
- **Consolidation (Months 2-4):** As new habits take root, blood sugar readings may improve. Some people notice reduced requirements for short-acting insulin or oral medications.
- **Assessment (Months 4-6):** Regular check-ins with your healthcare provider are essential. If blood glucose targets are consistently met, medication dosages may be safely reduced.
- **Sustained Progress (6 Months+):** Continued adherence to lifestyle changes can lead to further medication reductions, potentially leading to full remission for some individuals.

The Newcastle Remission Study

A powerful example comes from the UK's **Newcastle Remission Study**, which demonstrated that a calorie-controlled, whole-food diet led to remission in nearly half the participants. These individuals, some living with diabetes for over six years, were able to stop all medications as their blood sugar normalized. The study's success has inspired similar programs worldwide, from Scandinavia to Southeast Asia, each adapting the principles to local diets and customs.

Key Strategies for Reducing Medication

- **Work closely with your healthcare team:** Never stop or reduce medication without professional guidance. Your doctor will monitor your progress and adjust dosages safely.
- **Track your progress:** Use a glucose meter, food journal, or mobile app to identify what lifestyle changes have the greatest impact.
- **Prioritize sustainable habits:** Fad diets or extreme exercise regimens may yield quick results, but long-term success comes from consistency and balance.
- **Involve your support network:** Family, friends, or community groups can provide encouragement, accountability, and cultural adaptations that make change more enjoyable.

A Global Perspective

In India, where type 2 diabetes rates have soared alongside urbanization, community-based interventions focusing on traditional plant-based diets and group yoga have empowered thousands to reduce their medication needs. Similarly, programs in Australia's Indigenous communities embrace bush foods and physical activity rooted in cultural practices, reinforcing the idea that lifestyle change is most successful when it honors local customs and identities.

```
Memorable Fact: Sustained weight loss and healthy lifestyle changes can lead
to type 2 diabetes remission, allowing some individuals to maintain normal
blood sugar levels without medication.
Very Important: Always consult your healthcare provider before making any
changes to your diabetes medication regimen.
```

Reducing medication is not just a medical milestone; it's a testament to the body's remarkable capacity for healing. While not everyone will achieve complete medication independence, even modest reductions can mean fewer side effects, lower healthcare costs, and a renewed sense of control. In the next section, we'll discuss how to partner with your healthcare team to safely navigate these changes, ensuring your journey is guided by expert support and compassionate care.

10.4 Monitoring Progress Safely

As you begin to reduce your dependence on medication and embrace lifestyle changes, monitoring your progress becomes both a compass and a safety net. The process of reversing type 2 diabetes is dynamic—your body responds to changes in diet, exercise, and stress management, sometimes more quickly than anticipated. Close and consistent monitoring ensures you can celebrate progress, catch setbacks, and avoid the risks of overly rapid improvements, such as hypoglycemia.

Tools and Techniques for Tracking Health

Modern diabetes management offers a spectrum of tools for tracking your health, from traditional methods to the latest technology. The goal is to gain real-time insights into your blood sugar trends, medication needs, and overall well-being.

Blood Glucose Meters: Still a cornerstone for many, these devices allow you to check your blood sugar at home. Frequent testing—especially when adjusting medication or diet—can help spot patterns and prevent dangerous lows or highs.

Continuous Glucose Monitors (CGMs): More advanced, CGMs provide a steady stream of data, alerting you to fluctuations as they happen. These devices can be especially useful during periods of rapid change, such as when intensifying exercise or reducing medication.

Food and Activity Logs: Tracking what you eat and how much you move offers context for your numbers, helping you and your healthcare team identify what's working.

Blood Pressure and Weight Tracking: Since type 2 diabetes often coexists with hypertension and weight issues, monitoring these markers rounds out the picture of overall health.

Collaborative Monitoring: Partnering with Your Healthcare Team

No journey toward reversing type 2 diabetes is complete without the guidance of a supportive healthcare team. Regular check-ins with your doctor, diabetes educator, or pharmacist serve as milestones to reassess your plan and medication needs.

Schedule Regular Appointments: As you reduce medication, more frequent visits—sometimes every few weeks—may be necessary to review your numbers and adjust your regimen.

Share Your Data: Bring your glucose readings, food logs, and activity records to appointments. Transparency allows your provider to tailor recommendations and spot concerns early.

Ask Questions: If something feels off—a sudden dip in blood sugar, unexplained fatigue, or unusual symptoms—voice your concerns. Early intervention can prevent complications.

Real-World Story: Jamal's Journey to Empowerment

Jamal, a 52-year-old teacher from Kuala Lumpur, was initially overwhelmed by the prospect of reversing his diabetes. With his doctor's encouragement, he began tracking his progress with a simple spreadsheet, logging his meals, exercise, and glucose readings. When his numbers started to improve, his doctor gradually reduced his medication. One morning, after a particularly active weekend, Jamal noticed signs of hypoglycemia—shakiness and confusion. Because he had been diligently tracking his data, he recognized the warning signs and contacted his provider. Together, they adjusted his plan, ensuring a safer transition off medication. Jamal's commitment to monitoring did more than guide his recovery; it gave him confidence and independence.

The Role of Self-Reflection and Adjustment

Monitoring isn't just about numbers—it's about learning to listen to your body. Reflect regularly on how you feel: Are you more energetic? Sleeping better? Less thirsty? These subjective cues, when paired with hard data, provide a complete picture of your progress.

- **Notice Patterns:** Are blood sugar lows happening after intense exercise? Do certain foods spike your numbers?
- **Adjust Accordingly:** With your provider's guidance, use these insights to fine-tune your routine—perhaps adjusting meal timing, exercise intensity, or medication dose.

Global Perspective: Traditional and Modern Approaches

Across the world, people have blended modern and traditional approaches to monitoring progress. In Japan, for example, community health programs integrate technology with cultural practices, such as mindful eating and group exercise, to help people reverse diabetes safely. In rural India, community health workers visit homes to check blood sugar and blood pressure, ensuring even those with limited access to clinics can monitor their health.

These global efforts highlight a universal truth: regardless of setting, monitoring is central to sustainable, safe diabetes reversal.

Key Points to Remember

- **Monitor blood sugar frequently**, especially during medication changes.

- **Work closely with your healthcare team** for regular reassessment.
- **Be proactive**: Track food, activity, and subjective changes.
- **Learn from global perspectives** to enrich your own journey.

```
Reducing diabetes medication without close monitoring can lead to dangerous
low blood sugar (hypoglycemia)—always partner with your healthcare team to
adjust your plan safely.
```

Monitoring your progress isn't simply a medical task—it's an act of self-empowerment, a way to claim authority over your health journey. With careful tracking and collaborative support, you can navigate the transition away from medication safely and confidently

10.5 Integrating Traditional and Modern Medicine

Throughout history, people facing type 2 diabetes have sought healing in both **traditional remedies** and the innovations of **modern medicine**. Today, a growing number of individuals are discovering how integrating these two worlds—carefully and with medical guidance—can enhance their journey toward reducing medication dependency and achieving lasting health. This section explores how traditional practices and modern treatments can work together, highlights practical approaches, and shares real-world stories that illuminate this dynamic path.

Bridging Approaches: A Complementary Path

Modern medicine, with its arsenal of scientifically vetted medications and technologies, has transformed type 2 diabetes care. Yet, many traditional healing systems—like **Traditional Chinese Medicine (TCM)**, **Ayurveda** from India, and various Indigenous practices—have long histories of managing blood sugar and promoting wellness through food, herbs, movement, and mindfulness.

Rather than viewing these systems as mutually exclusive, a complementary approach can foster better outcomes. When thoughtfully combined, the best of both worlds may offer:

Personalized care, adapting strategies to suit individual needs and cultural values

Reduced medication dependency by supporting the body's natural regulation mechanisms

Enhanced psychological and emotional well-being from holistic practices

Modern Medicine: The Foundation

Modern medicine is grounded in rigorous research and evidence-based protocols. For many people, **oral hypoglycemic agents** (like metformin) or

injectable medications (such as GLP-1 agonists or insulin) are essential, especially at diagnosis or when blood sugar is dangerously high. These tools:

Reduce immediate health risks like hyperglycemia and diabetic complications
Offer reliable, measurable effects
Serve as a safety net while lifestyle changes take root

Yet, as we've explored, lifestyle interventions—improved diet, regular exercise, stress reduction—can reduce the need for lifelong medication.

Traditional Medicine: Ancient Wisdom

Various cultures have long used traditional remedies to manage diabetes symptoms:

Ayurvedic approaches utilize herbs like bitter melon, fenugreek, and gymnema, alongside dietary modifications and yoga, to balance blood sugar.
Traditional Chinese Medicine (TCM) employs herbal formulas, acupuncture, and tai chi to support pancreatic function and overall energy balance.
Indigenous North American practices sometimes incorporate plants like prickly pear cactus or blueberry leaves, combined with communal support and storytelling.

While scientific evidence varies for individual remedies, many traditional practices emphasize whole foods, movement, and stress reduction—core elements now recognized in mainstream diabetes care.

Real-World Example: India's Integrative Diabetes Clinics

In cities like Mumbai and Chennai, **integrative diabetes clinics** have become a model for combining modern and traditional care. Physicians and traditional healers work together, monitoring patients' blood sugar with modern diagnostics while offering yoga, meditation, and Ayurvedic dietary guidance. One patient, Arjun, shared how he began on two diabetes medications but, with regular yoga and herbal support, reduced his dosage under his doctor's supervision. "I feel more in control," Arjun notes, "because I'm treating my whole self, not just the numbers."

Navigating Integration: Best Practices

Successfully blending traditional and modern approaches requires clear communication and a team-based mindset:

- **Consultation and Honesty**: Always inform your healthcare provider about any herbs, supplements, or alternative therapies you use. Some can interact with medications or affect blood sugar unpredictably.
- **Evidence-Based Choices**: Seek traditional practices supported by research or long-standing safety records.
- **Monitoring and Adjustment**: Regularly track your blood sugar and medication needs as you add new practices. Adjustments should be made with medical supervision.

Key questions to consider:

- Does the traditional remedy have documented safety and efficacy?
- Is the practitioner experienced and reputable?
- How can the practice be incorporated without compromising modern treatment?

Global Perspective: The Case of Japan

Japan's approach to diabetes management often blends modern medicine with **Kampo**, its traditional herbal system. Many Japanese patients use Kampo remedies—under the guidance of both medical doctors and Kampo specialists—in conjunction with standard pharmaceuticals. This integrated model has inspired research collaborations and new clinical guidelines, offering a template for other countries seeking to harmonize care.

Cautions and Considerations

While integration can be empowering, it's vital to remain cautious:

- Not all "natural" remedies are safe or effective—some can disrupt blood sugar or interact dangerously with medications.
- Relying solely on traditional medicine in place of prescribed drugs can delay essential treatment and cause harm.
- Always approach integration as a supplement, not a substitute, for evidence-based medical management.

```
Type 2 diabetes is best managed with a team approach: combining the strengths
of modern medicine and traditional practices, under medical supervision, can
help reduce medication dependency and promote lasting health.
```

The journey to reverse type 2 diabetes is as much about honoring diverse traditions as it is about embracing innovation. By integrating the wisdom of the past with the tools of today, you can craft a care plan that is both effective and personally meaningful. In the next chapter, we'll explore how to solidify these gains, building habits and routines that support lifelong health and resilience—ensuring your progress is not just fast, but lasting.

10.6 Advocating for Your Health

Taking the reins of your health journey involves more than personal choices—it requires skillful communication and collaboration with your healthcare team. As you work to reduce medication dependency and optimize your diabetes management, becoming an effective self-advocate is essential. This not only empowers you, but also ensures your medical care is tailored to your unique needs, preferences, and progress.

Understanding Your Role in the Healthcare Partnership

The traditional model of healthcare often placed the patient in a passive role, receiving instructions from the doctor with little say in the process. Today, the most successful diabetes management stories come from those who see themselves as an active partner in their care. This means:

- **Asking questions** about medications, side effects, and alternatives.
- **Sharing updates** on your dietary changes, exercise routines, and blood sugar readings.
- **Expressing your goals**—for example, a desire to reduce or eliminate certain medications.
- **Requesting adjustments** to your care plan as your health improves.

This partnership is especially vital when striving for medication reduction. Your doctor may not be aware of the full extent of your lifestyle changes unless you communicate openly and consistently.

Preparing for Appointments: Making Every Minute Count

Medical appointments are often brief, so preparation is key. Consider these steps to maximize your time:

- **Track Your Progress:** Bring recent blood glucose readings, dietary notes, and an exercise log. This data shows tangible evidence of your efforts and helps guide the conversation.
- **List Questions and Concerns:** Write down anything you want to discuss, such as side effects, new symptoms, or interest in changing medications.
- **Review Medication List:** Note any non-prescription supplements or herbal remedies you're taking, as these can interact with diabetes drugs.

- **Set an Agenda:** Prioritize the most important issues you want to address, ensuring you leave the appointment with your questions answered.

Navigating Medication Reduction: A Collaborative Approach

Reducing or discontinuing diabetes medication should always be a medically supervised process. The sequence often follows a timeline like this:

- **Stable Blood Sugar Control:** After weeks or months of improved readings, your doctor may suggest reducing dosages.
- **Gradual Tapering:** Medications are reduced one at a time, with close monitoring.
- **Ongoing Assessment:** If blood sugar remains stable, further reductions may follow.

Throughout this process, your input is invaluable. Share any symptoms or challenges as dosages change. Remember, it's not uncommon for medication needs to fluctuate—what works now may need adjusting in the future.

Cultural Perspectives: Advocacy in Diverse Healthcare Settings

Healthcare systems vary dramatically around the world, shaping how people advocate for themselves. In Sweden, for example, patients are encouraged to participate in shared decision-making, an approach that has led to better diabetes outcomes and higher satisfaction rates. Contrast this with more hierarchical systems, where patients may feel hesitant to speak up. Regardless of cultural context, building confidence and learning to ask questions can bridge these gaps, ensuring everyone has the tools to pursue lasting health.

Overcoming Barriers to Advocacy

It's natural to feel intimidated when speaking with healthcare professionals, but remember: you are the expert on your body. To overcome common barriers:

- **Practice assertive communication:** Use "I" statements and express your needs clearly.
- **Bring a support person:** A friend or family member can help you remember details and provide encouragement.
- **Use reliable resources:** Equip yourself with evidence-based information to back up your questions.

The Power of Advocacy: Key Takeaways

Your voice matters in every health decision.

Effective self-advocacy can accelerate progress toward medication reduction. Building a partnership with your healthcare team leads to a more personalized and effective care plan.

Fact: Studies show that patients who actively participate in their healthcare decisions are more likely to achieve better glycemic control and report higher satisfaction with their treatment.

By advocating for your health, you are not only shaping your diabetes journey— you're setting a powerful example for others in your community and beyond. As you prepare to solidify your progress with lasting habits, remember that your partnership with healthcare professionals is a cornerstone of long-term wellness.

In the next chapter, we'll explore how to transform these changes into daily routines and rituals that reinforce your gains. Together, we'll build a strong foundation for a healthier, medication-independent future.

11 : Prevention – Stopping Diabetes Before It Starts

11.1 Identifying Prediabetes

Prediabetes is the crossroads where health decisions take on new urgency—a window of opportunity before the full onset of type 2 diabetes. Recognizing and understanding this condition is the first, crucial step in prevention. While prediabetes often goes unnoticed, its early identification can empower individuals to make meaningful changes that halt diabetes in its tracks.

What Is Prediabetes?

Prediabetes is a metabolic state where blood glucose levels are higher than normal, but not yet high enough to be classified as type 2 diabetes. It's akin to a traffic signal turning yellow—an alert to slow down and reassess your direction. The body's cells are becoming less responsive to insulin, a hormone essential for moving sugar out of the bloodstream and into cells for energy.

The Silent Progression

Prediabetes is often called a "silent" condition because it rarely causes symptoms. Most people with prediabetes are unaware of their risk until a routine blood test or a health crisis leads to a diagnosis. The lack of obvious symptoms makes regular screening critical, especially for those with risk factors such as:

- Family history of diabetes
- Overweight or obesity
- Sedentary lifestyle
- Age over 45
- Certain ethnic backgrounds (such as African American, Hispanic/Latino, Native American, Asian American, and Pacific Islander)
- History of gestational diabetes or polycystic ovary syndrome (PCOS)

Diagnostic Criteria: How Is Prediabetes Identified?

Medical professionals use several laboratory tests to identify prediabetes. Understanding these benchmarks helps demystify the process and encourages proactive health management. The most common tests include:

- **Fasting Plasma Glucose (FPG) Test:** Measures blood sugar after an overnight fast. Prediabetes is indicated by a result between 100 and 125 mg/dL.

- **Hemoglobin A1c (HbA1c) Test:** Reflects average blood sugar levels over the past two to three months. Prediabetes is defined as an A1c between 5.7% and 6.4%.

- **Oral Glucose Tolerance Test (OGTT):** Assesses blood sugar before and two hours after drinking a sugary beverage. Prediabetes is diagnosed if the two-hour value falls between 140 and 199 mg/dL.

It's important to note that a single abnormal result does not confirm prediabetes; repeat testing or additional evaluation is often recommended.

Why Early Identification Matters

Recognizing prediabetes is not simply about labeling a condition; it's about reclaiming agency over your health. Research from the **Diabetes Prevention Program** (DPP) in the United States demonstrated that individuals who identified as prediabetic and made modest lifestyle changes—losing just 5-7% of their body weight and engaging in regular physical activity—reduced their risk of developing type 2 diabetes by up to 58%.

Globally, similar programs have shown success. In Finland, for example, the **FIN-D2D** project mobilized communities to offer free screening events and culturally adapted lifestyle workshops, leading to measurable reductions in diabetes risk factors across diverse populations.

What to Do If You're at Risk

If you have risk factors or suspect you may have prediabetes, take the following steps:

- **Request Screening:** Ask your healthcare provider for blood sugar testing, especially if you're over 45 or have other risk factors.

- **Monitor Results:** Keep a personal health record of your glucose and A1c values.

- **Act Early:** Even small lifestyle tweaks can have a profound effect. Begin with manageable changes, such as adding a daily walk or substituting sugary drinks with water.

- **Follow Up:** Schedule regular check-ups to track your progress and adjust your prevention plan as needed.

Steps to Prevent Prediabetes

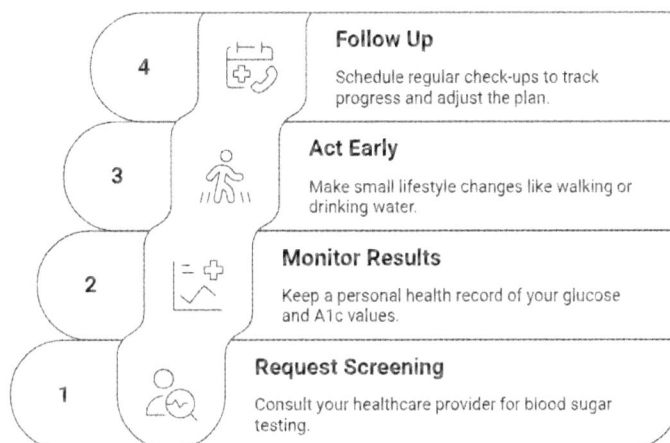

Follow Up
Schedule regular check-ups to track
progress and adjust the plan.

Act Early
Make small lifestyle changes like walking or
drinking water.

Monitor Results
Keep a personal health record of your glucose
and A1c values.

Request Screening
Consult your healthcare provider for blood sugar
testing.

```
Prediabetes can be reversed—lifestyle changes at this stage are more effective
than at any later point in preventing type 2 diabetes.
```

Awareness is the linchpin of prevention. Identifying prediabetes is not just a medical milestone; it's an invitation to reimagine your health journey. As we move forward, we'll explore practical strategies and lifestyle adjustments that can transform this knowledge into sustained, vibrant health—empowering you to stop diabetes before it starts.

11.2 Proven Prevention Strategies

As we step into the realm of prevention, it's essential to remember that **type 2 diabetes** is not an inevitable outcome—genetics may load the gun, but lifestyle pulls the trigger. The most compelling research consistently underscores the power of daily choices in shaping our health destiny. Prevention, then, is not a single act but a mosaic of intentional habits, each contributing to a future free of chronic disease.

The Pillars of Diabetes Prevention

Experts around the globe agree that a handful of core strategies are proven to reduce the risk of developing type 2 diabetes. These strategies are accessible, adaptable, and effective across cultures and backgrounds.

- **Balanced Nutrition**: Emphasizing whole foods, high fiber intake, and low glycemic index choices.
- **Regular Physical Activity**: Prioritizing both aerobic and resistance exercises.

- **Weight Management**: Achieving and maintaining a healthy body weight.
- **Stress Reduction**: Incorporating mindfulness, sleep hygiene, and social support.
- **Routine Health Monitoring**: Keeping tabs on blood sugar, blood pressure, and cholesterol levels.

Strategies for Diabetes Prevention

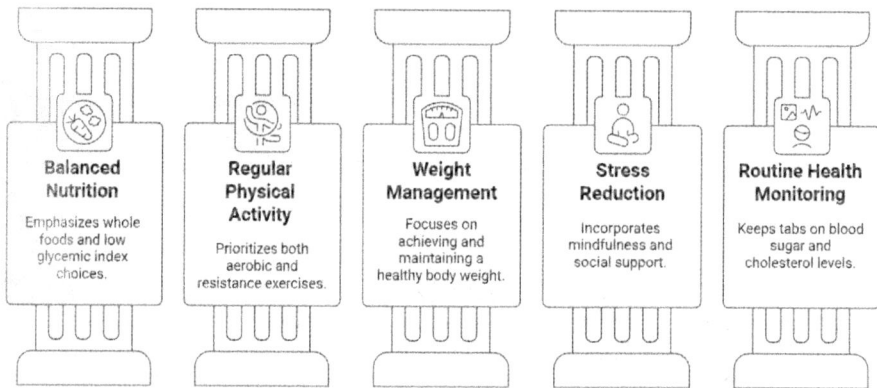

Balanced Nutrition	Regular Physical Activity	Weight Management	Stress Reduction	Routine Health Monitoring
Emphasizes whole foods and low glycemic index choices.	Prioritizes both aerobic and resistance exercises.	Focuses on achieving and maintaining a healthy body weight.	incorporates mindfulness and social support.	Keeps tabs on blood sugar and cholesterol levels.

Let's delve into each pillar, exploring the science and stories behind their success.

Balanced Nutrition: Building a Blood Sugar Buffer

A landmark study—the **Diabetes Prevention Program (DPP)** in the United States—found that participants who adopted a low-calorie, low-fat diet rich in fiber reduced their risk of developing type 2 diabetes by 58%. These results were even more pronounced among older adults, suggesting that it's never too late to benefit from dietary changes.

In the bustling streets of Mumbai, India, the **Mohan Diabetes Prevention Study** demonstrated similar success. Participants who replaced refined grains with lentils, whole grains, and local vegetables saw remarkable improvements in their blood sugar regulation. Their experience highlights the adaptability of prevention strategies to diverse cuisines and traditions.

Key nutrition habits include:

- Choosing whole grains over refined carbohydrates.
- Incorporating a rainbow of vegetables and fruits with a low glycemic index.

- Limiting added sugars and highly processed foods.
- Including healthy fats from nuts, seeds, and olive oil.

Physical Activity: Movement as Medicine

The DPP also underscored the transformative effect of regular exercise. Participants who engaged in at least **150 minutes of moderate activity per week**—such as brisk walking—experienced a profound drop in diabetes risk. Exercise enhances insulin sensitivity, aids weight loss, and supports cardiovascular health, forming a robust shield against type 2 diabetes.

A vivid example comes from Japan, where community-wide walking clubs have helped thousands of older adults maintain both physical and social well-being. In these groups, neighbors gather for daily walks, blending exercise with camaraderie—a winning combination for lasting health.

Practical exercise ideas:

- Brisk walking, cycling, or swimming.
- Strength training with weights or resistance bands.
- Yoga, tai chi, or other movement practices that build flexibility and reduce stress.

Weight Management: Small Changes, Big Impact

Even modest weight loss can have an outsized impact on diabetes prevention. The DPP found that losing just 5–7% of initial body weight—about 10–14 pounds for a 200-pound person—was enough to significantly lower diabetes risk. This finding is echoed in health systems worldwide, from the NHS in the UK to community clinics in Latin America.

Strategies for sustainable weight management:

- Setting realistic, incremental goals.
- Tracking progress with a journal or app.
- Seeking support from friends, family, or health professionals.

Stress Reduction: Protecting Your Pancreas

Chronic stress can disrupt hormones, raise blood sugar, and undermine efforts to eat well or stay active. Mindfulness-based techniques, such as meditation, deep breathing, and gratitude journaling, are increasingly recognized as essential tools in the prevention toolkit.

Consider the story of Maria, a schoolteacher in the Philippines. Facing the dual pressures of work and family, she began practicing ten minutes of guided meditation each morning. Over time, she noticed improved energy, steadier moods, and—confirmed by her doctor—better blood sugar readings. Maria's journey showcases the power of small, consistent acts of self-care.

Routine Health Monitoring: Staying Ahead

Regular check-ups allow for early detection and course correction. Monitoring fasting blood sugar, hemoglobin A1c, blood pressure, and cholesterol creates a feedback loop, encouraging proactive adjustments rather than reactive treatments.

Steps for effective monitoring:

- Schedule annual physical exams.
- Request relevant blood tests.
- Discuss results openly with your care team.
- Adjust your plan as needed based on data.

A Timeline for Prevention

Building Healthy Habits

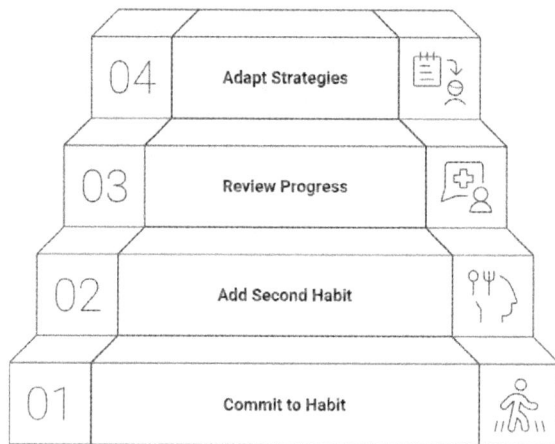

04	Adapt Strategies
03	Review Progress
02	Add Second Habit
01	Commit to Habit

- **Today**: Commit to one new habit—perhaps a daily walk or swapping white bread for whole grain.
- **One Month**: Build momentum by adding a second habit, like a weekly meal prep session or meditation practice.
- **Three Months**: Review your progress with your doctor and celebrate achievements.

- **Ongoing**: Adapt and refine your strategies as life evolves.

```
- Losing just 5-7% of your body weight can cut your risk of developing type 2
diabetes by more than half.
- Regular exercise—just 30 minutes five times a week—is as effective as many
medications in preventing type 2 diabetes.
```

Prevention is both a science and an art, shaped by evidence and enlivened by stories like Maria's and the walking clubs of Japan. By weaving these proven strategies into daily life, you can chart a course away from diabetes and toward robust, sustainable health. In the next section, we'll translate these principles into a step-by-step action plan—empowering you to take immediate, meaningful strides toward prevention and lifelong well-being.

11.3 Family and Cultural Prevention

Across the world, the food we eat, the activities we enjoy, and the habits we pass down through generations are shaped by family and culture. These influences can be powerful tools in the prevention of type 2 diabetes—or, if left unchecked, risk factors that quietly increase its prevalence. By understanding the impact of our familial and cultural environments, we can transform everyday moments into opportunities for lasting health.

The Family Table: Where Prevention Begins

For many, the family table is the heart of daily life, where values, stories, and recipes are shared. What we prepare and serve, the portions we dish out, and the rituals we follow often echo generations of tradition. In countries like **Japan**, for example, the practice of serving multiple small dishes—rich in vegetables, fish, and fermented foods— has long contributed to lower diabetes rates compared to nations with heavier, processed diets. In contrast, the rise of fast food and sugary beverages in **urban America** has coincided with a sharp increase in childhood obesity and type 2 diabetes.

Simple changes at home can make a world of difference:

- Swapping white rice or bread for whole grains at family meals
- Introducing more vegetables and legumes into stews, curries, and soups
- Celebrating fruit as a dessert instead of sugary treats
- Encouraging everyone to eat slowly and savor meals, honoring the body's natural cues for fullness

These shifts don't have to erase cherished traditions. Instead, they can adapt them—preserving cultural identity while fostering health.

Shared Activities: Movement as a Family Value

Physical activity is another area where family and culture intersect. In **India**, the tradition of morning walks in parks and neighborhoods is both a social and healthful practice. In the **Mediterranean region**, families often garden together or take evening strolls—a natural integration of exercise into daily life.

Building prevention into family routines can look like:

- Weekend nature hikes or bike rides instead of screen time
- Dance nights featuring music from your cultural heritage
- Organizing family sports, from soccer to traditional games

- Making movement a shared joy, rather than a chore, creates lifelong habits and memories.

The Power of Story: Breaking the Cycle

Family stories—both spoken and unspoken—shape our sense of what's possible. For many, a family history of diabetes can feel like a predetermined fate. Yet, as research now shows, **genes may load the gun, but lifestyle pulls the trigger**. Knowing the risks can be a catalyst for change, not resignation.

Cultural Shifts: Community as Prevention Partner

Communities shape what's accessible, affordable, and socially acceptable. In the **Pacific Islands**, for instance, rapid changes in diet and lifestyle, driven by globalization, have made type 2 diabetes a public health crisis. In response, local leaders in **Fiji** and **Samoa** are reviving traditional food cultivation and communal cooking practices that emphasize root vegetables and greens—reconnecting to ancestral wisdom as a means of prevention.

You can partner with your community to:

- Advocate for cultural events that feature healthy foods and active celebrations
- Support local farmers' markets or community gardens
- Share knowledge about diabetes prevention at churches, mosques, temples, or clubs

Key Family and Cultural Prevention Strategies

- Involve all family members—from children to grandparents—in meal planning and preparation.

- Respect and adapt cultural food traditions, making them healthier rather than abandoning them.
- Use family gatherings as opportunities for active play, not just eating.
- Talk openly about family health history and set shared wellness goals.
- Seek culturally competent healthcare advice that honors your background.

`Families who eat at least five home-cooked meals together per week have significantly lower rates of obesity and type 2 diabetes—across all cultures.`

Family and culture are the roots from which our health habits grow. By nurturing these roots with intention and knowledge, we can prevent type 2 diabetes from taking hold in future generations. In the next section, we'll bring these insights together with a practical, step-by-step action plan—empowering you to create sustainable change for yourself and your loved ones.

11.4 Case Studies from Around the Globe

In examining prevention strategies for type 2 diabetes, real-world stories and global case studies offer powerful illustrations of what works—and why. These narratives, drawn from diverse cultures and communities, show that while the path to prevention may vary, the core principles of lifestyle change, education, and community support remain universal. By exploring these examples, we gain a richer understanding of actionable measures and the potential for positive transformation, not just for individuals but for entire populations.

Finland's National Diabetes Prevention Program: A Model of Community Action

In the late 1990s, Finland faced a worrisome surge in type 2 diabetes cases, mirroring global trends. Rather than accept this as inevitable, Finnish health authorities launched the **Diabetes Prevention Study (DPS)**—a landmark initiative designed to test whether lifestyle changes could halt the disease in its tracks. The study enrolled individuals at high risk for type 2 diabetes, offering them personalized counseling on nutrition, exercise, and weight management.

The results were striking:

- Participants who adopted modest changes—such as losing 5% of their body weight, engaging in regular physical activity, and favoring whole grains and healthy fats—reduced their risk of developing diabetes by nearly 60% compared to the control group.
- These benefits persisted for years, proving that prevention is not only possible but sustainable.

The Finnish model went beyond individual willpower. Community-based workshops, peer support groups, and collaborations with schools and workplaces reinforced healthy behaviors at every level. This comprehensive approach transformed prevention into a collective effort, reshaping the national conversation about diabetes.

Key takeaways from Finland:

- Early intervention and education matter.
- Modest, achievable goals—like walking daily or swapping refined grains for whole grains—can have profound effects.
- Community engagement amplifies individual success.

India's Urban-Rural Divide: Adapting Strategies to Cultural Context

India, home to one of the world's fastest-growing diabetes populations, offers another compelling case study. Here, the challenge is twofold: tackling rising rates in urban centers while addressing unique risk factors in rural communities.

In metropolitan cities like Chennai, the **Diabetes Community Lifestyle Improvement Program (D-CLIP)** emerged as a culturally tailored intervention. Recognizing dietary patterns rooted in tradition, the program trained local health workers to deliver practical, relatable advice—like modifying classic Indian dishes to lower their glycemic index without sacrificing flavor. Group exercise classes were designed to be accessible and enjoyable, incorporating yoga and folk dance.

Meanwhile, in rural regions, prevention efforts focused on:

- Increasing awareness of diabetes symptoms, which often go unrecognized.
- Leveraging local leaders and trusted voices to combat stigma.
- Encouraging kitchen gardens and home-cooked meals over processed, packaged foods.

A key insight from India's experience is the importance of adapting prevention strategies to fit social norms, available resources, and cultural preferences. What works in an urban clinic may not resonate in a rural village—but both settings can achieve success with creativity and respect for local values.

Personal Story: Maria's Journey in Mexico

Maria, a 42-year-old mother of three from Oaxaca, Mexico, offers a deeply personal perspective on prevention. With a strong family history of type 2 diabetes, Maria was determined not to follow in her parents' footsteps. She began by attending local health workshops—initiatives supported by a partnership between Mexican authorities and international NGOs.

Maria learned to read food labels, cook traditional meals with less oil and sugar, and incorporate daily walks into her routine—even inviting neighbors to join her. Over the course of a year, she lost 15 pounds, lowered her blood sugar, and inspired a network of friends and family to make similar changes.

Maria's story underscores the ripple effect of individual action. Education and empowerment, when paired with community support, can break generational cycles and lay the foundation for healthier futures.

Lessons from Global Prevention Efforts

Across these stories, several themes emerge:

- **Empowerment through education**: Knowledge about nutrition, physical activity, and diabetes risk is a crucial first step.
- **Cultural adaptation**: Prevention strategies succeed when they honor local customs and address practical realities.
- **Community support**: Social networks—be they family, friends, or peer groups—provide essential encouragement and accountability.

These diverse experiences remind us that diabetes prevention is both a personal and a collective journey. By learning from global successes and challenges, we can tailor our own efforts to what truly works.

```
Fact: Research shows that lifestyle changes—such as losing just 5-7% of body
weight and increasing physical activity—can cut the risk of developing type 2
diabetes by more than half.
Very Important: Early intervention is key; the earlier healthy habits are
adopted, the greater the chance of preventing or delaying the onset of type 2
diabetes.
```

As we reflect on these global case studies, one message stands out: prevention is within reach, but it thrives on informed, culturally sensitive, and community-driven action. In the next section, we'll integrate these lessons into a step-by-step action plan—equipping you with the tools and confidence to prevent type 2 diabetes for yourself and your loved ones, no matter where you live.

11.5 Building a Culture of Wellness

Prevention of type 2 diabetes rarely happens in isolation. While individual choices matter, the environments in which we live, work, and socialize significantly influence our ability to maintain healthy habits. **Building a culture of wellness** means creating spaces—at home, in schools, workplaces, and communities—where making the healthy choice is the easy choice.

Consider the story of **Maria**, a teacher in Mexico City. When she learned she was prediabetic, Maria didn't just overhaul her diet and exercise routine—she rallied her colleagues to join her. Together, they started a lunchtime walking club and organized healthy potlucks. Within six months, the entire school noticed improved energy and fewer sick days. Maria's journey demonstrates that wellness can be contagious, and supportive networks can accelerate change.

The Ripple Effect: Wellness in Different Cultures

Globally, communities have developed unique approaches to health that can serve as inspiration. In **Japan**, the concept of "Ikigai"—a sense of purpose—encourages daily movement, strong social ties, and mindful eating. Okinawa's legendary longevity is partially credited to communal gardening and the practice of **hara hachi bu**—eating until 80% full. These traditions act as cultural guardrails, reducing the risk of chronic illnesses like type 2 diabetes.

Meanwhile, **Finland's North Karelia Project** offers a remarkable public health success story. In the 1970s, North Karelia faced soaring rates of heart disease and diabetes. Through community-wide campaigns, they shifted dietary habits, increased physical activity, and reimagined food environments. Over decades, chronic disease rates plummeted. This transformation wasn't just about education—it was about reshaping norms, making wellness part of local identity.

Creating Healthy Habits at Home

The foundation of a culture of wellness begins with the family unit. Small, consistent changes—shared meals, active weekends, limiting processed foods—create lasting impacts. Here are some approaches:

- Prioritize family meals with whole grains, lean proteins, and plenty of vegetables.
- Make physical activity a daily ritual, such as after-dinner walks or weekend bike rides.
- Involve children in grocery shopping and cooking to build lifelong healthy habits.
- Limit sugary snacks and drinks at home, making water the default beverage.

Workplaces as Wellness Hubs

Many adults spend the majority of their waking hours at work, making the workplace a crucial setting for diabetes prevention. Forward-thinking organizations have embraced wellness by:

- Instituting standing or walking meetings.
- Providing healthy cafeteria options and fruit baskets.
- Offering group exercise classes or gym memberships.
- Hosting stress-reduction workshops and mindfulness sessions.

When employers support wellness, they not only foster healthier employees but also improve productivity and morale.

Community Initiatives and Policy

Communities play a pivotal role in shaping health outcomes. Urban planners, local governments, and advocacy groups can promote wellness by:

- Building parks, playgrounds, and safe walking/biking paths.
- Organizing local farmers' markets for access to fresh produce.
- Launching public health campaigns on nutrition and physical activity.
- Supporting schools in providing balanced lunches and daily physical education.

When wellness is embedded in the fabric of a community, individual efforts are amplified by collective momentum.

Overcoming Barriers and Embracing Diversity

It's important to acknowledge that barriers to wellness—such as limited access to healthy foods, unsafe neighborhoods, or cultural norms—can make prevention challenging. Building a culture of wellness is not about imposing a single way of living but about leveraging strengths and traditions within each community.

For example, South Asian communities often gather for large family meals. By modifying traditional recipes—using brown rice instead of white, adding more vegetables, and reducing ghee—families preserve cultural identity while reducing diabetes risk. Inclusivity and respect for diversity are key to sustainable change.

Sustaining Momentum: A Timeline for Change

Creating a culture of wellness is a journey, not an overnight transformation. Here's a sample progression:

Journey to Wellness Culture

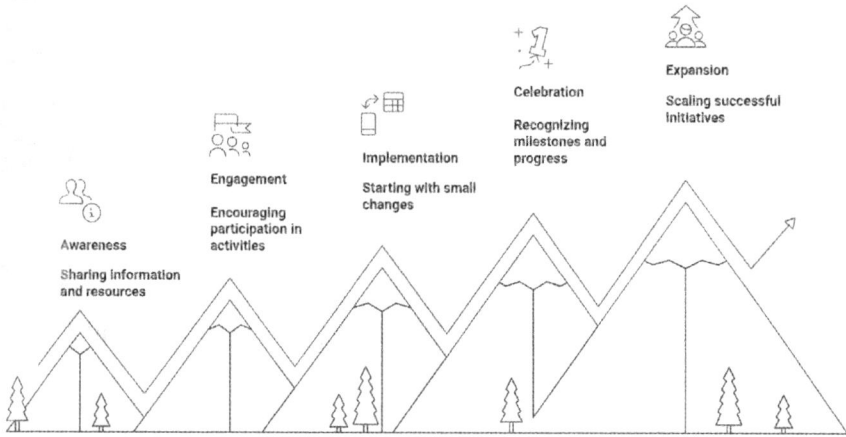

- **Awareness**: Share information and resources within families and communities.
- **Engagement**: Encourage participation in healthy activities and collective decision-making.
- **Implementation**: Start small, with one or two changes, and build on early successes.
- **Celebration**: Recognize milestones and share stories of progress.
- **Expansion**: Scale successful initiatives to involve more people and settings.

Type 2 diabetes prevention is most effective when healthy choices are woven into the fabric of daily life—at home, at work, and in the community. Supportive social networks and culturally relevant strategies are powerful drivers of lasting health.

A culture of wellness doesn't just protect us from type 2 diabetes; it enriches every aspect of our lives. When individuals, families, and communities come together in pursuit of health, prevention becomes not just possible, but inevitable. In the next section, we'll translate these insights into a practical, step-by-step action plan—empowering you to ignite change and safeguard your health for years to come.

11.6 The Power of Early Action

Early intervention is a critical turning point in the story of type 2 diabetes—a moment where the future can be rewritten with intention, knowledge, and decisive steps. For many, the first inklings of risk—perhaps a routine blood test showing elevated glucose or a family history whispering caution—offer a unique window of opportunity. Acting within this window, before symptoms deepen or complications arise, is not just wise; it's transformative. The power of early action lies in its ability to halt the progression of insulin resistance, restore the body's delicate metabolic balance, and prevent the cascade of health challenges that can follow unchecked diabetes.

Why Early Action Matters

Type 2 diabetes does not develop overnight. It is often preceded by a phase known as **prediabetes**, where blood sugar levels are higher than normal but not yet in the diabetic range. This stage is both a warning and a gift—a chance to intervene when the body is most receptive to positive change. Research shows that lifestyle changes made during prediabetes can prevent or even reverse the slide toward full-blown diabetes.

- **Greater reversibility:** Early in the disease process, the pancreas' insulin-producing cells have not suffered irreversible damage, making recovery more attainable.
- **Prevention of complications:** Acting early can prevent or delay complications such as heart disease, nerve damage, and vision loss.
- **Reduced medication dependence:** Timely lifestyle shifts can minimize or eliminate the need for lifelong pharmaceuticals.

A landmark study, the **Diabetes Prevention Program (DPP)**, demonstrated that individuals with prediabetes who adopted modest dietary changes and increased physical activity reduced their risk of developing type 2 diabetes by 58%. Among adults over 60, the risk dropped by a remarkable 71%. These numbers tell a story of hope—and underscore that the sooner the journey begins, the more dramatic the benefits.

The Global Perspective on Early Prevention

Globally, the imperative for early action is echoed across cultures and health systems. In Japan, for example, the government's **"Metabo" law** requires annual waist measurements for adults over 40, aiming to identify metabolic syndrome before it evolves into diabetes. Community interventions in rural India, meanwhile, focus on group exercise and locally grown vegetables to empower villagers at risk. These diverse approaches share a common thread: the recognition that timely intervention is the most powerful tool for prevention.

Steps to Seize the Window of Opportunity

The window for early action is often fleeting, but it is also full of promise. Here's how to capitalize on it:

- **Know Your Numbers:** Regular screenings for blood glucose, blood pressure, and cholesterol are essential, especially if you have a family history or belong to a high-risk group.

- **Understand the Warning Signs:** Fatigue, increased thirst, and frequent urination can signal rising blood sugar—even before a diagnosis.
- **Adopt Targeted Lifestyle Changes:**

    o Emphasize whole grains, fresh fruits, and vegetables.
    o Engage in at least 150 minutes of moderate activity per week.
    o Manage stress through mindfulness, yoga, or community support.

- **Build a Support Network:** Involve family, friends, or local groups for accountability and encouragement.
- **Consult Healthcare Professionals:** Early partnership with a doctor or nutritionist can personalize your prevention plan.

A Historical Anecdote: The Pima People

The story of the **Pima people** of Arizona is often cited in diabetes research. Historically, the Pima had low rates of diabetes, thanks to a physically demanding lifestyle and a diet rich in native plants. But as processed foods and sedentary habits replaced traditional ways, diabetes rates soared. Efforts to revive traditional foods and customs among younger generations have shown promise, highlighting that returning to time-tested habits—especially early in life—can powerfully counteract modern diabetes risk.

- **Early action** can halt or reverse the onset of type 2 diabetes.
- Lifestyle changes are most effective before the disease becomes entrenched.
- Community and cultural context shape both risk and response.

Fact: People with prediabetes who take early action can reduce their risk of developing type 2 diabetes by more than half.
Important: Once type 2 diabetes progresses, it becomes significantly harder to reverse—making early intervention crucial.

The stories of Maria, the Pima people, and global prevention programs remind us that early action is not about perfection, but about momentum and hope. By recognizing warning signs and responding with informed choices, anyone can dramatically alter their health trajectory. In the next section, we'll translate these insights into a practical, step-by-step action plan—empowering you to ignite change and safeguard your health for years to come.

12 : Real-World Success – Stories of Reversal and Resilience

12.1 The Journey to Diagnosis

For many, the path to a type 2 diabetes diagnosis is not sudden, but rather a gradual unveiling—an accumulation of subtle symptoms that are easy to dismiss or attribute to the hustle of daily life. **Fatigue**, frequent urination, unexplained thirst, and even minor changes in vision often arrive quietly, weaving themselves into routines until they become the new normal. Yet these early signals are the body's whispers, hinting at an underlying imbalance.

Consider the story of **Maria Sanchez**, a schoolteacher from Los Angeles. Maria lived a busy life, balancing her classroom duties with the joys and responsibilities of raising two children. She often found herself reaching for sugary snacks to boost her energy during long afternoons. Over months, she noticed her energy dips became more pronounced, and her visits to the restroom more frequent. Initially, she attributed these changes to stress and aging. It wasn't until a routine health screening at her school flagged elevated blood glucose levels that Maria began to piece together the puzzle. Her journey reflects the experience of millions worldwide: the slow realization that something fundamental has shifted.

A Timeline of Discovery

While each person's journey is unique, the sequence leading to diagnosis often follows a recognizable pattern:

- **Early Symptoms**

  o Subtle changes—such as persistent thirst, increased hunger, blurry vision, or tingling in the hands and feet—may emerge. These are easy to overlook or rationalize.

- **Escalating Concerns**

  o As symptoms intensify, individuals may experience unexplained weight loss or frequent infections. Family members might notice changes before the individual does.

- **Seeking Answers**

- o A decision is made to consult a healthcare provider, often prompted by a routine check-up or concern from loved ones.

- **Diagnostic Testing**

  - o Blood tests, including fasting glucose, oral glucose tolerance, and HbA1c, provide concrete evidence of elevated blood sugar levels.

- **Official Diagnosis**

  - o The confirmation brings a mix of emotions—relief at having answers, but also fear and uncertainty about the future.

- **The Turning Point**

  - o For many, this moment marks the beginning of a new chapter: learning, adapting, and ultimately reclaiming control over their health.

Globally, the journey to a type 2 diabetes diagnosis is shaped by cultural, social, and economic factors:

Access to Healthcare: In regions with limited resources, diagnoses are often delayed until complications arise.
Awareness and Education: Communities with strong health education programs tend to recognize symptoms sooner.
Cultural Norms: Dietary patterns, social expectations, and family history influence both risk and recognition.

These stories, whether from urban America or bustling India, highlight the universal challenges and opportunities in identifying type 2 diabetes early.

The Emotional Impact of Diagnosis

A diagnosis of type 2 diabetes is rarely just a medical event; it is an emotional crossroads. The news may trigger shock, denial, or even guilt—especially if there is a belief that lifestyle choices are solely to blame. Yet, as countless individuals have shown, this moment can also ignite a powerful resolve to change.

For Maria, the initial confusion gave way to determination. She sought out information, attended support groups, and connected with others facing similar journeys. For Rajiv, the diagnosis prompted reflection on his family traditions and a commitment to healthier choices—not just for himself, but for his children and grandchildren.

Type 2 diabetes can develop silently over years, with symptoms often dismissed until routine screening reveals the truth. Early detection is crucial: Lifestyle changes at this stage can dramatically improve outcomes and even lead to reversal.

The Power of Early Recognition

Recognizing the early signs of type 2 diabetes empowers individuals to take proactive steps. Timely diagnosis opens doors to interventions that can halt, and even reverse, disease progression. It's a reminder that, while the journey may begin with uncertainty, it can ultimately lead to transformation and resilience.

As we move forward, the next section will showcase how Maria, Rajiv, and many others embraced evidence-based strategies—from dietary changes to exercise routines—to not only manage, but actively reverse type 2 diabetes. Their stories illuminate the path from fear to hope, demonstrating that a diagnosis is not an end, but the start of a remarkable new chapter.

12.2 Taking the First Steps

The initial moments after a type 2 diabetes diagnosis can feel overwhelming—an emotional swirl of uncertainty, fear, and self-doubt. Yet, as the stories in this chapter reveal, the most powerful antidote to fear is action. Taking the first steps toward reversal is less about dramatic overnight transformations and more about a series of small, intentional choices. These choices, when woven together, become a tapestry of resilience and hope.

For many, the journey begins with a commitment: the decision not to be defined by a medical label, but to reclaim agency over one's health. This is where transformation takes root—when individuals choose to see their diagnosis as a call to action rather than a life sentence.

The First Steps: From Intention to Action

Every journey starts with a single step, and the path to reversing type 2 diabetes is no different. While the specifics will vary for each person, the foundational steps often include:

- **Self-Education:** Understanding what type 2 diabetes is, how it affects the body, and why lifestyle changes are so impactful.
- **Goal Setting:** Establishing realistic, attainable goals—whether it's reducing blood sugar levels, losing weight, or increasing daily activity.
- **Support Systems:** Reaching out to healthcare professionals, family, friends, or support groups for guidance and encouragement.

- **Dietary Adjustments:** Making conscious choices about what to eat, focusing on foods that support stable blood sugar.
- **Movement:** Incorporating regular physical activity, tailored to individual ability and interests.
- **Tracking Progress:** Using journals, apps, or simple logs to monitor food intake, activity, and blood sugar changes.

These steps are not meant to happen all at once. Instead, they unfold over time, becoming habits that create lasting change. The stories that follow illustrate how ordinary people, from diverse backgrounds, navigated these early days on their path to reversal.

Personal Story: Ravi's New Beginning

Ravi Patel, a 52-year-old teacher from Mumbai, received his diagnosis during a routine health check. The news shook him—both his father and uncle had struggled with diabetes-related complications. But rather than resign himself to the same fate, Ravi made a conscious decision to act.

- **Education:** Ravi spent hours reading about type 2 diabetes, seeking out reputable sources in English, Hindi, and Marathi. He learned about the glycemic index and how traditional foods could be adapted for better blood sugar control.
- **Support:** He joined a local walking group and enlisted his wife and children in meal planning, transforming the kitchen into a collaborative, health-focused space.
- **Diet:** Ravi replaced white rice with brown rice and experimented with lentil-based dishes, drawing on vegetarian traditions. He minimized sweets but allowed himself the occasional treat on festivals, balancing tradition and health.
- **Movement:** Daily walks became a family ritual, a time for bonding as much as for exercise.
- **Tracking:** Using a simple notebook, Ravi logged his meals, activity, and weekly blood sugar readings.

Within six months, Ravi's HbA1c (a measure of long-term blood sugar control) dropped from 8.2% to 6.1%. His story is a testament to the power of incremental change—and the importance of cultural and familial support in making new habits stick.

Historical Perspective: The Pima Community's Awakening

In the southwestern United States, the **Pima people** historically enjoyed robust health, sustained by a diet of beans, squash, corn, and wild game. However, the mid-20th century brought rapid lifestyle changes: processed foods replaced traditional diets, and physical activity declined. The result was one of the highest rates of type 2 diabetes in the world.

In response, community leaders and researchers began to revive traditional foodways and encourage movement through cultural dance and communal farming. Early adopters in the Pima community reported significant improvements—not only in blood sugar control, but also in overall well-being. This collective shift underscores the importance of reconnecting with heritage and leveraging community strengths in the journey to reversal.

Common First Hurdles—and How to Overcome Them

While each journey is unique, many face similar early challenges:

- **Skepticism or self-doubt:** It's normal to question whether meaningful change is possible, especially after years of ingrained habits.
- **Social pressures:** Navigating family gatherings, cultural festivals, or work events can be daunting.
- **Information overload:** The sheer volume of advice—sometimes conflicting—can breed confusion.

Overcoming these hurdles often means:

Starting small, celebrating every victory, no matter how minor.
Seeking out allies, whether in family, faith communities, or online support groups.
Focusing on progress, not perfection.

```
Fact: Even modest weight loss—just 5-10% of body weight—can dramatically
improve insulin sensitivity and blood sugar control in people with type 2
diabetes.
Important: The journey to reversal is not linear; setbacks are normal, but
persistence is what leads to lasting change.
```

Taking the first steps requires courage, curiosity, and a willingness to embrace both triumphs and setbacks. As Ravi's journey and the Pima community's revival show, lasting health is built on a foundation of small, consistent actions—supported by knowledge, culture, and community. In the next section, we'll explore how these early efforts blossom into sustained success, examining strategies for maintaining progress and preventing relapse on the road to lasting health.

12.3 Sustaining Change

For many people, the initial diagnosis of type 2 diabetes is a wake-up call that triggers meaningful change. The path to reversal is rarely a straight line; rather, it is a journey of resilience, adaptation, and the steady accumulation of small victories. But what happens after the first wave of motivation passes? How do individuals move from early successes—such as losing weight, lowering blood glucose, or reducing medication—to a way of living that supports ongoing health?

The stories of those who have reversed type 2 diabetes often reveal that sustaining change is both a personal and communal process. After the initial momentum fades, it is the formation of new habits, the support of others, and the development of a resilient mindset that carry people forward.

Building Habits That Last

Sustaining change requires more than willpower. Research and lived experience show that lasting transformation hinges on the development of daily routines that become almost automatic over time.

- **Routine and Ritual:** Establishing consistent meal times, regular exercise sessions, and daily mindfulness practices helps anchor healthy behaviors. Simple rituals—like a morning walk or preparing a nutritious breakfast—become pillars of a new lifestyle.
- **Environmental Cues:** People who succeed in sustaining change often modify their environments to reduce temptation and promote healthier choices. This might include keeping healthy snacks visible, planning meals ahead, or removing sugary foods from the home.
- **Tracking and Reflection:** Many successful individuals keep journals or use digital apps to track blood sugar, activity levels, and food intake. This reflection enables early identification of patterns and potential pitfalls, so adjustments can be made before setbacks occur.

The Case of Maria: A Habitual Transformation

Maria, a 52-year-old schoolteacher from Mexico City, was diagnosed with type 2 diabetes in her late forties. Her early efforts—motivated by fear—were successful, but she soon realized that to sustain her progress, she needed more than motivation. Maria began batch-cooking healthy meals on Sundays with her family, turning it into a shared ritual. She joined a local walking group, finding camaraderie and accountability. Over time, her healthy habits became second nature, and her diabetes remained in remission for over five years.

The Power of Community Support

Social support is a common thread in many reversal stories. Whether through family, friends, support groups, or online communities, connecting with others who understand the journey provides encouragement and accountability.

- **Peer Support:** Sharing struggles and successes with others battling diabetes fosters resilience and reduces feelings of isolation.
- **Cultural Adaptation:** In many cultures, food is a central aspect of gatherings. Those who succeed often find creative ways to adapt traditional recipes, ensuring that their health goals align with their cultural and social lives.

A Global Example: The United Kingdom's NHS Diabetes Prevention Programme

The United Kingdom's **NHS Diabetes Prevention Programme** is a powerful example of community-driven change. Participants receive group-based support, nutrition education, and exercise guidance. Studies have shown that those enrolled in the program experience greater success in sustaining lifestyle changes than those who go it alone. The shared journey—rooted in local community and collective accountability—translates into higher rates of long-term diabetes remission.

Navigating Setbacks and Preventing Relapse

Even the most successful individuals experience setbacks—holidays, stressful life events, or unexpected health issues can derail progress. The key to sustaining change is not perfection, but resilience.

- **Anticipate Triggers:** Understanding personal triggers—such as emotional eating or social pressures—helps individuals plan coping strategies in advance.
- **Reframe Setbacks:** Instead of viewing lapses as failures, resilient people see them as learning opportunities and recommit to their goals.
- **Ongoing Education:** Staying informed about diabetes management and new research empowers individuals to make informed decisions and adapt as needed.

Timeline: Sustaining Change Over Time
- **Initial Change (Months 1-3):** Motivation is high, and dramatic dietary and lifestyle adjustments are possible.
- **Habit Formation (Months 4-12):** New behaviors become routine; support structures and rituals form.

- **Resilience and Adaptation (Year 2 and beyond):** Setbacks may occur, but strong habits and social support enable quick recovery and continued progress.

The Role of Identity and Purpose

Perhaps most importantly, many who achieve lasting change report a shift in self-identity. They no longer see themselves as "a diabetic," but as someone who chooses health daily. This profound transformation often serves as the ultimate anchor for long-term success.

```
Memorable Fact: Studies show that individuals who maintain at least a 7%
weight loss and engage in 150 minutes of moderate exercise per week can reduce
their risk of diabetes relapse by over 50%.
```

Sustaining change is an ongoing process that blends habit, support, and resilience. The real-world examples in this chapter make clear that while the journey may be challenging, it is possible—and deeply rewarding—to transform one's life after a diabetes diagnosis. As we move forward, the next section will focus on practical tools and resources you can use to build your own support network and continue your journey toward lasting health.

12.4 Global Voices of Success

Across continents and cultures, the journey to reverse type 2 diabetes is as varied as the people who undertake it. While the science of blood sugar regulation is universal, the stories of transformation are deeply personal and shaped by context—by food traditions, social support, health care systems, and individual resolve. In this chapter, we step out of the clinic and into the real world, where everyday people are rewriting their futures through courage, discipline, and hope. Their voices echo the enduring truth: diabetes may be a global epidemic, but solutions are as diverse as humanity itself.

Maria's Path: Tradition Meets Transformation in Mexico

Maria, a 54-year-old grandmother from Oaxaca, Mexico, received her diagnosis of type 2 diabetes after years of feeling fatigued and increasingly reliant on sweetened beverages common in her community. Initially, the news felt overwhelming. Yet Maria's story is a testament to the intersection of cultural tradition and evidence-based change.

Her journey began by revisiting her roots. Instead of processed foods and sugary drinks, Maria turned to the time-honored staples of her region: beans, corn tortillas, squash, and leafy greens. Drawing on advice from a local clinic's diabetes educator, she learned about the **glycemic index** and began to substitute high-glycemic foods with more complex carbohydrates native to her area. Family meals became opportunities for collaboration—her children joined her evening walks, and her husband experimented with preparing nopales (cactus paddles) as a fiber-rich side dish.

Maria's progress over twelve months was remarkable:

- **Month 1:** Swapped sodas for homemade hibiscus tea without added sugar; began tracking blood sugar.
- **Month 3:** Integrated brisk daily walks with her grandchildren as a family routine.
- **Month 6:** Attended community cooking classes focused on traditional, low-glycemic recipes.
- **Month 12:** Reduced her medication under her doctor's supervision after consistently improving her A1C results.

Maria's story illustrates how blending cultural heritage with scientific guidance can foster not only personal health but also community resilience. Her transformation rippled outward—her neighbors, inspired by her success, began to adopt similar changes, demonstrating the contagious power of positive example.

Rajiv's Resilience: A Tech Worker's Journey in India

On the other side of the globe, Rajiv, a 39-year-old IT engineer in Bengaluru, India, faced a mounting health crisis. Long hours at his desk, combined with a diet heavy in refined carbohydrates and convenience foods, led to a diagnosis that threatened his career and quality of life.

Rajiv's approach was shaped by both technology and tradition. With the encouragement of his physician, he started using a continuous glucose monitor and a smartphone app to track his meals and activity. But he also drew upon his family's vegetarian culinary heritage, exploring dishes centered on lentils, chickpeas, and a variety of regional vegetables.

His reversal timeline unfolded as follows:

- **Week 1:** Began daily walks during lunch breaks; replaced white rice with brown rice and millet.
- **Month 2:** Joined an online support group for Indian professionals managing diabetes.
- **Month 4:** Adopted a weekly yoga and meditation routine to address work-related stress.
- **Month 9:** Blood sugar levels stabilized; his doctor reduced his medication dosage.

Rajiv's greatest insight was the realization that sustainable change stemmed from adapting modern tools to his unique cultural and occupational context. His story underscores the value of digital health resources and peer support, especially in fast-paced urban environments.

A Historical Perspective: The Pima People's Turning Point

The struggle with type 2 diabetes is not new; history offers powerful lessons. Among the Pima people of the American Southwest, rates of type 2 diabetes soared in the 20th century as traditional diets gave way to processed foods. However, recent decades have seen a revival of ancestral foodways—beans, squash, tepary beans, and wild greens—paired with increased physical activity.

Community-led initiatives have demonstrated that returning to time-tested foods and movement can restore health and hope, even in populations disproportionately affected by diabetes. This historical shift highlights the importance of cultural context and the enduring wisdom embedded in traditional lifeways.

Key Lessons from Global Stories

- **Cultural food traditions** can be powerful allies in diabetes reversal when paired with modern knowledge.
- **Family and community support** magnifies individual efforts, creating a ripple effect of wellness.
- **Technology and peer networks** offer new avenues for accountability and encouragement.
- **Historical context** reminds us that the roots of health are often found in the past, waiting to be reclaimed.

Sustainable diabetes reversal is most successful when individuals blend modern science with personal and cultural strengths—making every victory unique, yet universally inspiring.

The journeys of Maria, Rajiv, and the Pima community remind us that reversing type 2 diabetes is neither a solitary endeavor nor a one-size-fits-all process. Their stories illuminate the immense value of connecting personal motivation with cultural wisdom and modern tools. As we move to the next section, we will explore practical resources and strategies—ranging from support groups to digital apps—that can help you build your own network of encouragement and accountability, paving the way for lasting health.

12.5 Lessons Learned

As we reflect on the remarkable journeys of individuals who have faced type 2 diabetes head-on and emerged healthier, several key lessons emerge. These real-world stories aren't just tales of personal triumph—they are blueprints for sustainable change, offering hope and guidance to anyone seeking to reclaim control over their health. The following insights distill the wisdom gained from these diverse experiences, demonstrating that reversal is not only possible, but achievable with determination, support, and the right strategies.

Patterns of Success

Across continents and cultures, people who have successfully reversed or managed type 2 diabetes share common threads in their stories. Their paths may differ in detail, but the principles are strikingly similar:

- **Consistency over Perfection:** Instead of aiming for flawless adherence to every guideline, successful individuals focus on steady, incremental progress. They embrace slip-ups as learning opportunities, not failures.
- **Support Systems Matter:** Whether through family, community groups, online forums, or professional coaching, those who thrive rarely do it alone.
- **Personalization Is Key:** No single dietary or exercise plan works for everyone. Tailoring strategies to fit cultural preferences, daily routines, and unique body responses is essential.
- **Holistic Mindset:** True reversal goes beyond blood sugar readings. It involves emotional resilience, self-compassion, and a focus on overall well-being—not just numbers.

Stories That Inspire

Let's revisit two very different, yet equally inspiring, stories that illuminate the diversity and universality of the diabetes reversal journey.

1. Maria's Mediterranean Turnaround

Maria, a 58-year-old teacher living in southern Italy, was diagnosed with type 2 diabetes after constant fatigue and blurred vision. At first, she felt overwhelmed by the dietary restrictions and feared losing the culinary heritage she cherished—olive oil, fresh bread, and homemade pasta.

Instead of abandoning her roots, Maria worked with a nutritionist to adapt her traditional Mediterranean diet. She replaced white bread with whole-grain artisanal loaves, increased her intake of legumes and leafy greens, and learned to savor smaller portions of pasta. Regular walks along the coastline became her daily ritual, reducing stress and strengthening her resolve.

Within eighteen months, Maria's HbA1c levels had normalized, and her doctor celebrated her medication-free status. Maria's journey underscores the power of adapting evidence-based principles within familiar cultural frameworks, proving that managing diabetes doesn't mean sacrificing identity.

2. James's Community-Driven Comeback

In a bustling city in South Africa, James, a 45-year-old accountant, learned of his diabetes diagnosis after a routine company health screening. Initially, he kept the news private, fearing stigma. But his turning point came when he joined a local community center's diabetes support group, where he met others facing similar challenges.

James began tracking his meals with a smartphone app and joined weekly group exercise classes. The camaraderie and accountability of his peers kept him motivated, even when progress felt slow. Over two years, James lost over 20 kilograms, improved his cardiovascular fitness, and gradually reduced his reliance on medication.

James's story highlights the profound impact of community—how collective encouragement can transform individual resolve into lasting change.

Historical Perspective: An Evolving Understanding

The concept of reversing type 2 diabetes isn't new, but its acceptance has evolved over time. In the mid-20th century, diabetes was widely viewed as an irreversible, progressively worsening disease. However, landmark studies in the past 20 years—such as the DiRECT trial in the United Kingdom—have challenged this narrative, demonstrating that significant weight loss, dietary intervention, and comprehensive lifestyle changes can induce remission in a substantial proportion of patients.

This shift from resignation to possibility has empowered individuals and clinicians alike, ushering in a new era of proactive, patient-centered care.

Key Takeaways for Lasting Health

From these stories and the collective wisdom of the diabetes community, several transformative lessons emerge:

- **Start Where You Are:** You don't need to overhaul your entire life overnight. Begin with small, manageable changes and build from there.
- **Seek Support:** Harness the power of community, whether through family, friends, or digital networks.
- **Honor Your Culture:** Adapt healthy habits to fit your own traditions, tastes, and preferences.
- **Track Progress, Not Perfection:** Celebrate improvements, no matter how incremental, and learn from setbacks.

- **Prioritize Mental Well-being:** Stress management, self-compassion, and emotional resilience are as vital as nutrition and exercise.

Nearly half of individuals who achieve significant weight loss through dietary and lifestyle changes can put type 2 diabetes into remission, according to major clinical studies.

Effective diabetes reversal is not about deprivation, but about creating sustainable, enjoyable habits that fit your life.

The stories and lessons shared in this chapter illuminate the path from diagnosis to vibrant health. Real-world examples reveal that with perseverance, support, and culturally sensitive strategies, lasting change is within reach for people everywhere. As we move forward, the next chapter will guide you through practical resources and step-by-step strategies to help you create your own personalized action plan—empowering you to turn inspiration into transformation on your journey to lasting health.

12.6 Celebrating Milestones

Transformation rarely happens overnight. For many living with type 2 diabetes, the journey toward reversal and lasting health is marked by a series of small, meaningful victories. Celebrating these milestones—no matter how minor they may seem—plays a pivotal role in maintaining motivation, reinforcing positive behaviors, and fostering a sense of agency. Each step forward is a testament to resilience, determination, and the unwavering belief that change is possible.

Rosa's Triumph: Reclaiming Life, One Step at a Time

Consider the story of **Rosa Mendoza**, a retired schoolteacher in Mexico City. Diagnosed with type 2 diabetes in her early sixties, Rosa faced a future clouded by medication, fatigue, and the constant fear of complications. At first, the changes seemed insurmountable. But with the support of her family and guidance from her doctor, she began to make small, sustainable adjustments.

She swapped white rice for fiber-rich black beans in her daily meals.
She made a habit of walking through her neighborhood park every morning.
She practiced mindful eating, paying attention to portions and savoring her meals.

At first, progress was incremental. But Rosa kept a journal of her achievements, however small: a lower morning blood sugar reading, a brisker walk, a new healthy recipe tried. Each entry became a celebration—a reminder that her efforts mattered.

After six months, Rosa's doctor delivered remarkable news: her HbA1c levels had dropped into the prediabetes range, and her need for medication was reduced. Over the next year, she was able to discontinue medication entirely under medical supervision. Rosa's journey was not defined by a single, dramatic turning point, but by a series of milestones—each one celebrated, each one fueling her resolve.

The Science of Positive Reinforcement

Why is celebration so crucial? Research in behavioral psychology shows that **positive reinforcement**—acknowledging achievements, no matter how minor—strengthens new habits and makes it more likely they will endure.

Key benefits of celebrating milestones include:

- Boosting self-confidence and self-efficacy.
- Reducing feelings of overwhelm by focusing on progress rather than perfection.
- Encouraging consistency through emotional rewards.
- Creating a feedback loop that makes healthy behaviors more enjoyable.

From Mumbai to Melbourne: Diverse Journeys, Shared Triumphs

Success stories span the globe. In **Mumbai, India**, 45-year-old Rajesh Singh faced a similar journey. Raised on a diet rich in refined carbohydrates and deep-fried snacks, Rajesh's diagnosis came as a shock. Inspired by a local diabetes education initiative, he joined a community walking group and began experimenting with traditional recipes that incorporated whole grains and fresh vegetables.

Rajesh celebrated each milestone—walking 5,000 steps a day, preparing a new healthy dish, sharing his story with others. Over time, his efforts translated into measurable improvements: lower fasting glucose, renewed energy, and a sense of purpose. The community celebrated Rajesh's achievements, making each victory a shared triumph.

Practical Ways to Celebrate Your Wins

Celebration doesn't have to mean grand gestures. Often, the most meaningful rewards are those that connect you to your deeper motivations and values. Here are some practical, culturally adaptable ways to honor your progress:

- Share your achievement with a supportive friend, family member, or online community.
- Treat yourself to a non-food reward—such as a new book, a relaxing outing, or a favorite activity.
- Reflect on your journey in a gratitude journal, noting what you've learned and how you've grown.

- Volunteer to mentor someone else beginning their diabetes reversal journey.
- Mark the occasion with a symbolic gesture—planting a tree, lighting a candle, or creating a piece of art.

Timeline: Celebrating Milestones on the Path to Reversal
- **Week 1:** First healthy meal swap; log your experience.
- **Week 2:** Achieve a week of daily walks; share your accomplishment.
- **Month 1:** Noticeable drop in fasting glucose; reward yourself with a small gift.
- **Month 3:** HbA1c improvement; celebrate with friends or family.
- **Month 6 and beyond:** Medication reduction or discontinuation; reflect on your transformation and set new goals.

Celebrating milestones isn't about perfection—it's about progress. Each step forward, no matter how small, brings you closer to your vision of lasting health.

```
Fact: Studies show that individuals who track and celebrate small health
achievements are more likely to sustain long-term lifestyle changes and
achieve diabetes remission.
Important: Reversal is a journey; every positive change counts and deserves
recognition.
```

As we have seen through Rosa's and Rajesh's stories—and through countless others around the world—reversing type 2 diabetes is not a solitary act, but a series of shared, celebrated milestones. Acknowledging these achievements transforms the journey from a burden into a source of pride and joy. In the next chapter, we'll explore how to turn inspiration into action with practical resources and strategies to craft your personalized path to lasting health. Let's take the next step—together.

13 : Building Lasting Habits – Tools for Sustainable Health

13.1 The Psychology of Habit Change

Lasting change begins in the mind. For anyone seeking to reverse type 2 diabetes, the **psychology of habit change** is foundational. Far beyond willpower or fleeting motivation, habits shape the daily decisions that collectively determine our health. Understanding how habits work, why they form, and—most importantly—how to change them is essential for sustainable progress on the journey to lasting health.

At the core, a **habit** is an automatic behavior triggered by a specific cue and rewarded with a sense of satisfaction or relief. Think of the morning cup of coffee, the evening walk, or even the seemingly innocuous biscuit with afternoon tea. Over time, these routines become ingrained, quietly influencing blood sugar, energy, and overall well-being.

The Habit Loop: Cue, Routine, Reward

Habits form through a three-part process often called the **habit loop**:

- **Cue**: A trigger, such as a time of day, emotional state, or place, prompts the behavior.
- **Routine**: The behavior itself—grabbing a snack, skipping a workout, or choosing a healthy meal.
- **Reward**: The payoff, which could be pleasure, relief, or a sense of accomplishment.

For example, consider **Martha**, a retired teacher from Chicago. Every evening after dinner, she would reach for a sugary dessert—her cue was the end of the meal, the routine was eating dessert, and the reward was comfort and enjoyment. When Martha was diagnosed with type 2 diabetes, she realized that this nightly habit was spiking her blood sugar. By recognizing her cues and swapping her routine for a healthier alternative—like a bowl of berries or herbal tea—she still enjoyed her reward, but in a way that supported her health goals.

The Science Behind Changing Habits

Research shows that changing habits is less about fighting old patterns and more about **replacing** them. The brain craves the reward, not necessarily the routine itself. By keeping the cue and reward but altering the behavior, new, healthier habits can take root.

- **Start Small**: Trying to overhaul your life overnight is rarely sustainable. Focus on one manageable change at a time—swapping white rice for brown, adding a daily 10-minute walk, or meditating before bed.
- **Consistency Is Key**: Habits are built through repetition. The more often you repeat a new routine, the more automatic it becomes.
- **Track Progress**: Journaling or using a habit-tracking app can reinforce accountability and highlight successes.

Cultural and Global Perspectives on Habit Change

Different cultures have long traditions of habit formation and change. In **Japan**, the practice of **kaizen** (continuous improvement) encourages making small, incremental changes daily, a philosophy that has transformed workplaces and individual lives. In India, the practice of **yoga** and mindful eating rituals helps many people become more conscious of their food choices and stress responses—critical elements for diabetes management.

Worldwide, communities are proving that sustainable change is possible by blending cultural values with modern science. For instance, a diabetes reversal program in the United Kingdom integrated traditional cooking classes with behavioral coaching, empowering participants to adapt familiar recipes and routines, resulting in significant improvements in blood sugar control.

Overcoming Barriers and Staying Motivated

Changing habits is rarely a smooth journey. Obstacles—stress, social pressures, or setbacks—are inevitable. What sets successful habit changers apart is their resilience and flexibility.

- **Anticipate Challenges**: Identify triggers that may lead to unhealthy choices and plan alternative responses.
- **Build a Support Network**: Share your goals with friends, family, or a support group. Social accountability can be a powerful motivator.
- **Celebrate Small Wins**: Recognizing progress, no matter how minor, fuels motivation and confidence.

A Personal Story: Raj's Journey

Raj, a software engineer in Bangalore, struggled with erratic eating habits and late-night work sessions. After his diagnosis, Raj worked with a health coach to identify his cues—work stress and fatigue—and gradually replaced his evening fast food with home-cooked, low-glycemic meals. Over several months, Raj not only lost weight but also significantly reduced his reliance on medication. His story illustrates that, with the right strategies and support, even deeply ingrained habits can be transformed.

```
Fact: Research shows that it takes an average of 66 days to form a new habit—
consistency matters more than perfection.
Very Important: The most successful diabetes reversals come from sustainable,
not extreme, lifestyle changes.
```

The journey to lasting health is not about perfection, but persistence. By harnessing the psychology of habit change, you can build daily routines that steadily move you toward reversing type 2 diabetes. Remember, every small, positive choice adds up over time, creating momentum for lifelong wellness.

As we move to the next section, we'll explore **practical tools and resources** that support your new habits—ensuring you have the structure and guidance needed to thrive. The foundation is set; now, let's build the framework for sustainable results.

13.2 Making Healthy Choices Automatic

At the heart of sustainable health change lies an often-underestimated force: **habit**. Habits are the routines and behaviors we perform, often unconsciously, that shape our daily lives. For those working to reverse type 2 diabetes, making healthy choices automatic means transforming conscious, sometimes difficult decisions into effortless routines. When you no longer have to debate whether to choose a salad over fries, or whether to go for a brisk walk after dinner, you free up mental energy for other aspects of life—and set yourself up for long-term success.

Research in behavioral science shows that habits are formed through a **cue-routine-reward loop**. You encounter a cue (like waking up in the morning), perform a routine (drinking a glass of water), and receive a reward (feeling refreshed). Over time, this loop becomes ingrained, and the behavior happens with little thought.

The Science of Automaticity

Automaticity is the process by which a behavior becomes automatic. According to studies from University College London, it takes an average of 66 days to form a new habit, but the timeline can vary greatly depending on the complexity of the behavior and individual differences. The key is **repetition** in the same context.

For diabetes management, this means:

Consistently choosing foods with a low glycemic index for each meal
Establishing a regular exercise schedule
Monitoring blood sugar at set times each day

By repeating these actions in a stable context, your brain begins to associate specific cues—like mealtime or waking up—with healthy routines.

Tools to Build Automatic Healthy Choices

Building automaticity doesn't happen overnight, but several tools can accelerate the process:

Building Automatic Healthy Choices

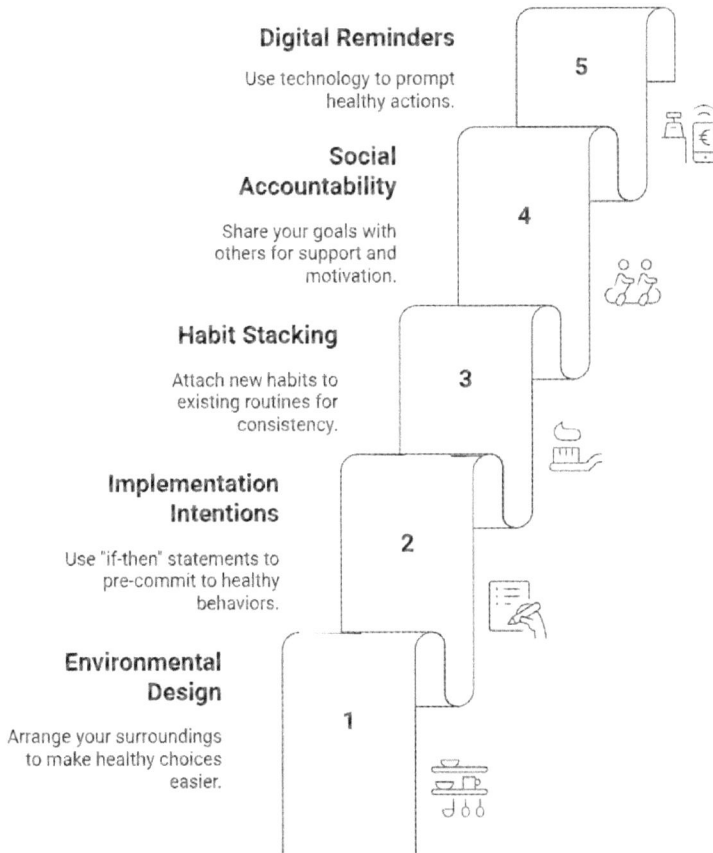

Digital Reminders
Use technology to prompt healthy actions.
5

Social Accountability
Share your goals with others for support and motivation.
4

Habit Stacking
Attach new habits to existing routines for consistency.
3

Implementation Intentions
Use "if-then" statements to pre-commit to healthy behaviors.
2

Environmental Design
Arrange your surroundings to make healthy choices easier.
1

- **Environmental Design:** Make healthy choices the easy choices by arranging your environment. Stock your fridge with fresh produce, keep a water bottle at your desk, and remove sugary snacks from your pantry.
- **Implementation Intentions:** Use "if-then" statements to pre-commit to healthy behaviors. For example, "If I feel stressed after work, then I will take a 10-minute walk before dinner."

- **Habit Stacking:** Attach new habits to existing routines. If you already brush your teeth every night, add a habit of stretching or preparing your breakfast for the next day right afterward.
- **Social Accountability:** Share your goals with friends or join a support group. Knowing others are aware of your commitment can reinforce your resolve.
- **Digital Reminders:** Use smartphone alarms or apps to prompt healthy actions, such as drinking water or checking your blood sugar.

Historical Perspective: The Okinawan Approach

In Okinawa, Japan, one of the world's "Blue Zones" known for longevity and low rates of chronic disease, healthy habits are deeply woven into daily life. The traditional Okinawan saying "**hara hachi bu**"—which means "eat until you are 80% full"—is a cultural cue that shapes eating behaviors. Meals are built around vegetables, legumes, and small portions of fish, and regular movement is part of the community's rhythm. These habits aren't enforced by willpower; rather, they are reinforced by environment and culture, making them automatic and sustainable.

Overcoming Obstacles

Even with the best intentions, obstacles will arise. Stress, social events, or unexpected changes in routine can disrupt new habits. The key is to anticipate these challenges and have a plan:

Identify Triggers: Recognize situations that tempt you to revert to old habits, such as late-night snacking or skipping exercise.

Plan Alternatives: If you can't make it to the gym, have a home workout ready. If dining out, review the menu in advance for healthy options.

Show Self-Compassion: Acknowledge setbacks as part of the process. One missed step does not erase your progress.

Making It Last

The journey to reversing type 2 diabetes is not about perfection, but about consistency. Celebrate small victories, track your progress, and remember that healthy habits are an investment in your future self. Over time, what once required effort will become as automatic as tying your shoes.

```
Forming a new habit takes, on average, two months of consistent repetition—so
patience and persistence are key.
Surrounding yourself with healthy cues and supportive community increases your
chances of long-term success.
```

In summary, making healthy choices automatic is about harnessing the power of habit to simplify daily decisions and empower lasting change. By designing supportive environments, leveraging cues, and embracing cultural wisdom, you lay the groundwork for sustainable health. As we move forward, let's explore how tracking your progress and celebrating milestones can further fuel your journey to lasting wellness—one habit at a time.

13.3 Tracking and Accountability

Consistent tracking transforms intention into action. For many who embark on the path to reverse type 2 diabetes, the difference between fleeting efforts and lasting change often hinges on their ability to observe, measure, and reflect on daily choices. Self-monitoring brings an empowering sense of control—turning vague goals like "eat healthier" or "exercise more" into concrete, measurable steps.

Why does tracking matter? Research consistently demonstrates that people who monitor their habits—whether it's food intake, physical activity, or blood sugar levels—are more likely to stick to their goals and achieve better health outcomes. Recording this information makes progress visible, highlights patterns, and reveals areas for adjustment. It's not about judgment or perfection, but about developing self-awareness and celebrating small victories.

Consider the story of **Ana**, a schoolteacher from Brazil. After her type 2 diabetes diagnosis, Ana started jotting down her meals and glucose readings in a notebook. Within weeks, she noticed that her blood sugar spiked after certain traditional dishes. By making small changes—like swapping white rice for beans and whole grains—she saw steady improvements. For Ana, the act of tracking became a daily ritual, transforming her relationship with food and her sense of agency over her health.

Tools and Techniques for Effective Tracking

In today's world, tracking your health habits can be as simple or as sophisticated as you want. The key is to choose tools and methods that fit seamlessly into your lifestyle and feel sustainable.

- **Pen and Paper Journals:** Some people, like Ana, prefer the tangible act of writing. Journals make it easy to jot down not just meals and numbers, but also moods, energy levels, and reflections.
- **Mobile Apps:** Digital tools such as MyFitnessPal, Glucose Buddy, or Apple Health allow for real-time tracking and graphical feedback. These apps can sync with wearable devices, making it easier to log steps, sleep, and glucose levels.

- **Wearable Devices:** Fitness trackers and continuous glucose monitors (CGMs) provide instant feedback and allow for trend analysis over days, weeks, or months.
- **Community Platforms:** Online forums and support groups offer shared tracking templates and group challenges, adding a sense of camaraderie and accountability.

Cycle of Health Habit Tracking

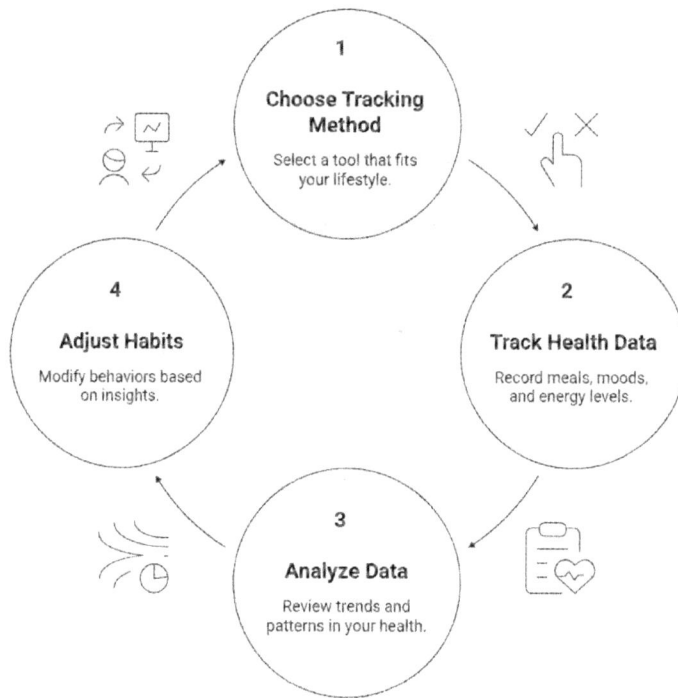

The most effective tracking system is the one you'll actually use. Some enjoy the structure of daily logs, while others prefer weekly check-ins. The important thing is to make it a regular habit—integrated into your routine, not an afterthought.

Making Accountability Work for You

Accountability is the invisible force that turns personal goals into public commitments. When you share your intentions with others, you invite encouragement, support, and—sometimes—a gentle nudge when motivation wanes.

- **Buddy System:** Pair up with a friend, family member, or fellow traveler on the diabetes reversal journey. Share goals, check in regularly, and celebrate each other's wins.

- **Professional Guidance:** Health coaches, dietitians, or diabetes educators can offer expert feedback, personalized strategies, and structured follow-up.
- **Group Challenges:** Join or create group initiatives—like a 30-day low-glycemic meal plan or a daily steps challenge. Friendly competition and collective goals can boost engagement and make the process more enjoyable.

Let's look at the experience of **Michael**, a retiree from South Africa. Michael joined a local walking group after his diagnosis. The group met three times a week, and members tracked their steps using pedometers. Knowing he'd be missed if he skipped a session, and seeing his progress alongside others, kept Michael motivated—long after his initial enthusiasm faded. Within six months, not only had he lost weight and improved his blood sugar control, but he'd also built a supportive community around his new lifestyle.

Overcoming Common Barriers

Despite the benefits, tracking and accountability can feel overwhelming at first. Here are some strategies to overcome common obstacles:

Overcoming Tracking Obstacles

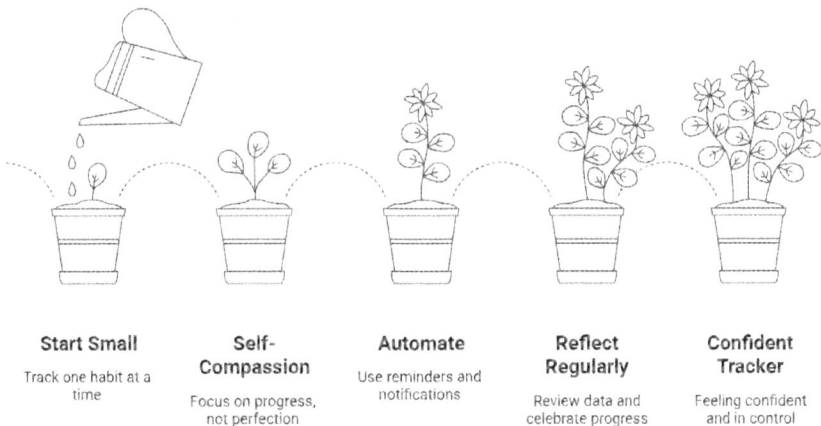

Start Small	Self-Compassion	Automate	Reflect Regularly	Confident Tracker
Track one habit at a time	Focus on progress, not perfection	Use reminders and notifications	Review data and celebrate progress	Feeling confident and in control

- **Start Small:** Begin by tracking just one habit—like daily blood sugar or breakfast choices. Add more as you gain confidence.
- **Be Kind to Yourself:** If you miss a day or make a mistake, avoid self-criticism. Focus on progress, not perfection.

- **Automate When Possible:** Use reminders, alarms, or app notifications to prompt daily check-ins.
- **Reflect Regularly:** Take a few minutes each week to review your data. Celebrate improvements and identify areas for gentle adjustment.

Remember, tracking is a tool for insight and empowerment—not a test to pass or fail.

```
- Consistent self-monitoring of blood glucose, diet, and activity levels is
linked to improved diabetes management and higher rates of remission.
- Accountability, whether through social support or professional guidance,
significantly boosts long-term adherence to healthy habits.
```

Tracking and accountability are the scaffolding that supports your journey to lasting health. By making your efforts visible and enlisting the support of others, you transform hope into habit—and setbacks into stepping stones. As you become more skilled at observing and celebrating your progress, you'll find that sustainable change becomes not just possible, but inevitable.

In our next section, we'll delve into strategies for **celebrating progress and overcoming setbacks**, ensuring you stay resilient and motivated, no matter where you are on your path to reversing type 2 diabetes. Let's continue building the foundation for a healthier, more empowered future—one mindful step at a time.

13.4 Community and Social Support

Type 2 diabetes is often described in terms of numbers—A1C levels, milligrams of glucose, or pounds lost—but the journey to reversing it is deeply human. While individual determination is crucial, research and real-life stories consistently show that **community and social support** are among the most powerful predictors of lasting health change. When we feel supported, understood, and connected, our motivation soars, our ability to overcome setbacks improves, and healthy habits are much more likely to stick.

Why Social Support Matters

Humans are inherently social beings. Our behaviors, beliefs, and even our biology are shaped by the people around us. In the context of reversing type 2 diabetes, support can come in many forms:

- **Emotional encouragement** during difficult days
- **Accountability** partners to keep goals on track
- **Practical advice** about meal planning or exercise routines
- **Celebration of successes**, no matter how small

A robust support network not only lifts our spirits but also reduces stress—a key factor in blood sugar regulation. Studies have shown that those who engage in diabetes support groups, community classes, or even online forums have better long-term outcomes than those who attempt lifestyle changes alone.

Real-World Example: The "Blue Zones" Approach

One inspiring global example comes from the **Blue Zones**—regions of the world with the highest concentration of centenarians and low rates of chronic diseases, including type 2 diabetes. In places like Okinawa, Japan, and Nicoya, Costa Rica, community is woven into daily life. Families cook together, neighbors walk in groups, and social gatherings revolve around shared healthy meals.

In Okinawa, the concept of **moai**—a lifelong circle of friends who support each other through joys and hardships—has been credited with reducing stress and promoting healthy behaviors. Members of a moai help one another stay accountable to healthy routines, offer emotional support, and create a sense of belonging. These practices have been linked to significantly lower rates of type 2 diabetes and cardiovascular disease compared to Western countries.

Building Your Support Structure

Not everyone has a ready-made moai, but everyone can cultivate meaningful support. Here's how to build your own network for lasting health:

- **Identify Your Allies:** Start with family, friends, coworkers, or neighbors who are supportive of your health journey. Share your goals and ask for their encouragement.
- **Seek Out Support Groups:** Local hospitals, diabetes clinics, and community centers often offer group classes or support meetings. These provide a safe space to share experiences and learn from others facing similar challenges.
- **Leverage Online Communities:** Digital forums, social media groups, or virtual meetups can connect you with people worldwide. These resources can be especially helpful if you live in a rural area or prefer the anonymity of online interaction.
- **Join Activity-Based Groups:** Walking clubs, cooking classes, or gardening groups offer the added benefit of social engagement while promoting healthy lifestyle habits.
- **Enlist Professional Support:** Dietitians, diabetes educators, and counselors can become trusted partners on your journey. Don't hesitate to ask your healthcare provider for referrals.

Cultural Perspectives on Support

Social support is expressed in diverse ways across cultures. In many African and South Asian communities, extended families often live together and share meals, naturally creating opportunities for collective healthy eating and activity. In the United States, faith-based organizations and churches frequently offer health ministries, walking groups, and communal meals that foster both spiritual and physical well-being.

These global perspectives remind us that support can take many forms—formal or informal, in-person or virtual—but the underlying principle remains the same: **we thrive together**.

Making Support Sustainable

Building and maintaining your support system requires intentionality:

- **Communicate regularly:** Check in with your support network, even when things are going well.
- **Express gratitude:** A simple thank you strengthens bonds and encourages ongoing support.
- **Be a supporter, too:** Offering encouragement to others reinforces your own commitment.

Fact: Individuals with strong social support are up to 50% more likely to achieve long-term diabetes remission compared to those without consistent support.
Very Important: Chronic stress and isolation can raise blood sugar levels, making community connections a vital part of diabetes management.

Reflection and Transition

Harnessing the power of community transforms your journey from a solitary struggle into a shared mission. Whether through family, friends, peer groups, or cultural traditions, social support is the glue that helps healthy habits become second nature. As we move forward, let's explore how to track your progress and celebrate each achievement—turning your path to health into a story of lasting success.

13.5 Adapting to Life Transitions

Life's only constant is change. Whether it's a new job, moving to a different city, the arrival of a child, or even the unexpected loss of a loved one, transitions are an inevitable part of the human experience. For individuals managing or reversing type 2 diabetes, these moments can be pivotal. They can threaten hard-won progress or, conversely, act as catalysts for deeper commitment to health. Understanding how to adapt your healthy habits to shifting circumstances is essential for lasting success.

Recognizing the Impact of Transitions

When routines are disrupted, even the most disciplined individuals can feel off-balance. The stress of change can easily sideline health priorities, leading to skipped meals, poor food choices, missed exercise sessions, or neglected blood sugar monitoring. Yet, transitions also offer a chance to reassess and reinforce what matters most.

Take the story of **Maria**, a schoolteacher from São Paulo, Brazil. After being diagnosed with type 2 diabetes, Maria adopted a Mediterranean-style diet and daily walking routine. Things went smoothly until her school transferred her to a night shift. The schedule upheaval threatened her meal planning, sleep, and exercise. Instead of succumbing to frustration, Maria turned her challenge into an opportunity—enlisting her coworkers in healthy meal prepping and organizing lunchtime walks. These small adaptations helped her maintain her health gains and inspired her peers to join her wellness journey.

Strategies for Navigating Change

Successfully managing diabetes through life's transitions requires flexibility, planning, and a willingness to seek support. Consider these key strategies:

Anticipate Disruptions: Before a major transition, brainstorm potential obstacles to your routine and prepare solutions. For example, if you're moving, research grocery stores or fitness centers near your new home.

Prioritize Non-Negotiables: Identify the 2-3 core habits critical to your diabetes management—such as daily glucose checks, a balanced breakfast, or evening walks—and commit to maintaining them, no matter what.

Leverage Social Support: Changes can feel isolating; reach out to friends, support groups, or online communities for encouragement and accountability.

Use Technology: Apps for meal planning, glucose tracking, or virtual workouts can help you stay connected to your goals, even on the go.

Practice Self-Compassion: Setbacks are normal during transitions. Avoid all-or-nothing thinking; each day is a new opportunity to recommit.

A Global Perspective: Tradition Meets Transition

Across cultures, adapting healthy habits through transitions is a universal challenge. In India, where family gatherings and festivals are often centered around food, newly diagnosed diabetics may find festive seasons daunting. Yet, some communities have embraced adaptation by reimagining traditional dishes—reducing sugar, swapping refined grains for whole ones, or adding more vegetables—to align with diabetes-friendly guidelines. These creative shifts honor heritage while supporting health, illustrating that adaptation does not require abandoning cultural identity.

Creating Your Personal Transition Toolkit

To prepare for the inevitable changes life brings, consider building a **transition toolkit**:

- **List Your Essential Habits:** Write down the daily or weekly actions that most impact your blood sugar and wellbeing.
- **Identify Vulnerable Points:** Think about which habits are most likely to be challenged during times of change.
- **Develop Backup Plans:** For each vulnerable habit, create a simple backup plan. For example, if you can't cook at home, identify two healthy takeout options.
- **Communicate Needs:** Let those around you know about your health priorities and enlist their support.
- **Reflect and Adjust:** After each transition, spend a few minutes reflecting— what worked, what didn't, and what could be improved next time?

Personal Story: The Power of Resilience

Consider **David**, a retiree in England who reversed his type 2 diabetes through plant-based eating and regular cycling. When his wife became ill, David's priorities shifted overnight. He found himself overwhelmed, his routines upended by caregiving duties. At first, David slipped back into old eating habits. However, recalling his previous success, he reached out to a local diabetes support group. The encouragement and practical tips he received helped him reestablish routines, this time with new flexibility— shorter, more frequent exercise sessions, and preparing simple, nutritious meals in bulk. David's experience demonstrates that resilience and adaptation are as crucial as knowledge in the journey toward lasting health.

```
Fact: During periods of high stress or major life transitions, blood sugar
levels can fluctuate more than usual, making self-monitoring and flexible
routines even more vital for diabetes management.
```

Transitions need not derail your progress. Instead, by embracing change, planning ahead, and seeking support, you can transform challenges into stepping stones toward greater health. As you continue your journey, remember that lasting habits are not about perfection—they're about persistence, flexibility, and self-compassion.

In the next section, we'll explore how to track your progress and celebrate milestones, turning your ongoing efforts into a narrative of achievement and resilience. This approach not only reinforces your commitment but also reveals the remarkable story of your health transformation.

13.6 Preventing Relapse

Relapse is not a sign of failure—it's a common and often expected part of the process when working to reverse type 2 diabetes. Even the most diligent individuals can find themselves slipping back into old habits, especially during times of stress, celebration, or disruption to daily routines. Recognizing this reality, and preparing for it, is crucial for long-term success.

Type 2 diabetes management isn't a sprint; it's a lifelong journey. There will be days when temptations seem overwhelming, or when motivation wanes. Understanding that these moments do not erase your progress but are simply bumps on the road empowers you to respond with resilience rather than regret.

Common Triggers for Relapse

Several factors can contribute to a relapse in healthy habits:

- **Emotional Stress:** Life changes, loss, or anxiety can lead to comfort eating or skipping routines.
- **Social Situations:** Holidays, family gatherings, or cultural events often center around food and drink.
- **Travel and Holidays:** Changes in schedule and environment can disrupt meal planning and exercise.
- **Fatigue and Burnout:** The ongoing effort of lifestyle change can sometimes feel exhausting, leading to lapses.
- **Complacency:** Feeling "cured" or symptom-free may tempt you to relax your diligence.

By identifying these triggers, you can develop strategies to navigate them, ensuring that a temporary setback doesn't become a lasting reversal.

Building Resilience: Strategies to Prevent Relapse

Successful, sustainable health is built not just on initial changes, but on your response to challenges along the way. Here are practical tools to help you stay on track:

- **Reflect and Reframe:**

  - Instead of self-blame, view relapses as opportunities for learning. Ask yourself: What triggered this lapse? How did I feel? What could I do differently next time?

- **Revisit Your Motivation:**

- Regularly remind yourself of the reasons you chose this path—be it your family, your dreams, or the desire for a fuller, more active life. Visual cues, such as photos or affirmations, can help keep your motivation front and center.

- **Plan for High-Risk Situations:**

  - Prepare for challenging scenarios in advance. If you know a celebration is coming, plan your meals ahead, bring a healthy dish, or decide to take a walk after eating.

- **Build a Support Network:**

  - Share your journey with friends, family, or a support group. Accountability partners and community support can make a remarkable difference in staying motivated and feeling understood.

- **Develop Coping Skills:**

  - Learn non-food ways to manage stress, such as meditation, gentle exercise, or creative hobbies.

- **Track Your Progress:**

  - Use journals, apps, or charts to monitor your blood sugar, meals, and activity. Seeing your achievements in black and white can be a powerful motivator.

- **Forgive Yourself Quickly:**

  - If you slip, don't dwell on guilt. Acknowledge it, reset your intentions, and continue forward.

Historical Perspective: The Pima People

The Pima people of Arizona have one of the highest rates of type 2 diabetes in the world, a stark contrast to their ancestors, who thrived on a traditional diet of beans, squash, and corn and maintained active lifestyles. When modern processed foods and sedentary living entered their community, diabetes rates soared. Today, Pima health advocates are working to revive ancestral eating and activity habits, teaching that relapse is a communal challenge, not just an individual one. Their story underscores the importance of societal support and cultural identity in preventing relapse and sustaining health.

Key Reminders in Preventing Relapse

Consistency over perfection: It's your overall pattern, not individual lapses, that shapes your health.

Every day is a new opportunity: You can always choose to restart, no matter how many times you've stumbled.

```
Relapse is a normal part of lifestyle change—what matters most is your
response, not the setback itself.
Regular self-reflection and community support are powerful tools for getting
back on track after a lapse.
```

Preventing relapse is about more than willpower; it's about building a resilient mindset, cultivating support, and planning for real-life challenges. Both personal stories and broader historical lessons remind us that setbacks can be stepping stones to deeper understanding and lasting change. With these tools, you are well-equipped to navigate the ups and downs of your journey, reinforcing the habits that lead to lasting wellness.

14 : A New Beginning – Your Path to Lasting Health

14.1 Reflecting on Your Progress

As you reach this pivotal point in your journey, pausing to reflect on your progress is more than a pat on the back—it's an essential step in solidifying lasting change. Managing and potentially reversing type 2 diabetes isn't a sprint; it's a marathon of mindful choices, resilience, and learning. By taking stock of your achievements, setbacks, and the road ahead, you not only celebrate your growth but also uncover fresh motivation to sustain your health.

Measuring Success Beyond Numbers

Many people equate progress with test results: lower fasting glucose, improved HbA1c, or a shrinking waistline. While these are vital indicators, your journey encompasses much more. Consider the habits you've built, the knowledge you've gained, and the sense of control you now wield over your health. These intangible victories often matter most in the long run.

> **Behavioral changes**: Have you made exercise a regular part of your week? Are whole foods now staples in your kitchen?
>
> **Mindset shifts**: Do you approach meals with curiosity instead of fear? Have you found strength in setbacks, using them as learning opportunities?
>
> **Quality of life**: Are your energy levels higher? Do you feel more confident discussing your condition with loved ones or healthcare providers?

Every step forward, however small, is worth acknowledging.

Charting Your Journey: A Timeline Approach

Let's break down your progress into a simple timeline to help you appreciate the distance you've covered and identify where you might want to focus next.

- **Weeks 1-2**: Initial adjustments—cutting down on sugary snacks, reading food labels, and perhaps experiencing the first dip in cravings or blood sugar swings.
- **Weeks 3-6**: Settling into routines—experimenting with new recipes, fitting in regular walks or gym sessions, and noticing subtle improvements in mood or sleep.
- **Months 2-4**: Tangible changes—significant drops in blood glucose, weight loss, and perhaps a conversation with your doctor about reducing medication.

- **Months 5 and beyond**: Mastery and maintenance—handling holidays, social gatherings, and stress without derailing your health; inspiring others through your story.

As you revisit this timeline, remember that everyone's path is unique. Some experience quick improvements, while others see steady, gradual progress.

Stories of Triumph: Real-World Reflections

Consider the story of **Carlos**, a chef from Mexico City who was diagnosed with type 2 diabetes at age 54. Initially overwhelmed, Carlos gradually adapted his cooking style—swapping white rice for quinoa, loading dishes with colorful vegetables, and experimenting with herbs instead of salt and sugar. Within six months, not only did his HbA1c levels drop, but he also inspired his extended family to embrace healthier eating. Carlos's journey underscores the importance of cultural adaptation and shows that healthful changes need not erase cherished culinary traditions.

Or take **Anita**, a schoolteacher in Mumbai, who decided to tackle her diagnosis with a community-driven approach. She joined a local walking group, incorporated traditional plant-based dishes with lower glycemic loads, and used WhatsApp to share recipes and encouragement with her peers. Anita's success reminds us that social support and cultural relevance can make lifestyle changes more sustainable and joyful.

Recognizing Setbacks as Stepping Stones

Progress is rarely linear. Fluctuating blood sugar, busy workweeks, or tempting holiday spreads can lead to setbacks. Instead of viewing these as failures, see them as necessary learning moments. Each misstep offers insight: What triggers old habits? Which support systems help you rebound? By reflecting honestly and compassionately, you set the stage for stronger, more lasting change.

Simple Tools for Ongoing Reflection

To make reflection a practical part of your routine, consider the following strategies:

Journaling: Keep a daily or weekly log of your meals, activity, emotions, and blood sugar readings. Over time, patterns will emerge.

Progress check-ins: Schedule monthly self-assessments—or, if you prefer, check-ins with a healthcare provider or support group.

Celebrate milestones: Mark significant achievements, whether it's a new cooking skill, a completed exercise challenge, or a successful medication reduction.

The Science of Sustained Success

Research consistently shows that **self-monitoring**—regularly tracking your behaviors and outcomes—dramatically improves the likelihood of reversing type 2 diabetes and maintaining these gains. When you reflect, you become an active participant in your health, rather than a passive recipient of medical advice.

```
Memorable Fact: Studies show that individuals who regularly reflect on their
behaviors and outcomes are up to 50% more likely to maintain long-term
diabetes remission.
```

Moving Forward with Confidence

Reflecting on your progress is not a one-time task but an ongoing practice. Each step, each reflection, builds a foundation for lasting change. Your story, like those of Carlos and Anita, is still being written. As you continue this journey, remember that setbacks are part of the process, and every victory—big or small—deserves recognition.

In summary, embracing reflection cements your achievements, deepens your self-awareness, and fuels your resilience. As you turn the page to the next chapter, you'll discover how to set sustainable goals and harness your progress for lifelong health. The journey is ongoing, and your new beginning is only just unfolding.

14.2 Setting New Goals

As you embark on this chapter of renewal, the foundation you've built—through learning, self-reflection, and daily habit changes—sets the stage for the most critical step yet: **setting new goals**. These goals serve not just as benchmarks of progress, but as beacons to guide your next steps, carrying you from short-term victories to a lifetime of health and empowerment.

Why Goals Matter in Diabetes Reversal

Goals are more than wishful thinking; they are commitments to yourself. In the context of **type 2 diabetes reversal**, setting clear and actionable goals has been shown to:

Foster accountability and motivation
Offer measurable milestones for tracking progress
Transform abstract wishes ("I want better health") into actionable realities ("I will walk 30 minutes every morning")
Help navigate setbacks with resilience and perspective

A study published in the journal *Diabetes Care* demonstrated that individuals who set and monitored personalized health goals were significantly more likely to achieve sustained glycemic control and reduce medication dependency than those who did not.

The act of goal-setting turns intention into action and marks the difference between fleeting change and lasting transformation.

Crafting SMART Goals for Diabetes Management

Vague ambitions are easy to ignore, but **SMART goals**—Specific, Measurable, Achievable, Relevant, and Time-bound—provide clarity and structure. Let's break this down with an example:

Refining Goals for Diabetes Management

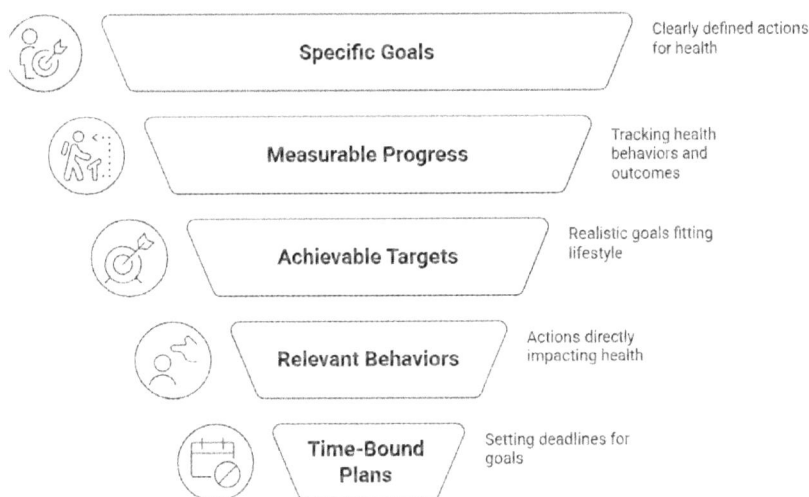

Specific Goals — Clearly defined actions for health

Measurable Progress — Tracking health behaviors and outcomes

Achievable Targets — Realistic goals fitting lifestyle

Relevant Behaviors — Actions directly impacting health

Time-Bound Plans — Setting deadlines for goals

- **Specific:** Instead of "I will eat healthier," try "I will include at least two servings of non-starchy vegetables at lunch and dinner."
- **Measurable:** Track your progress by keeping a food and activity journal.
- **Achievable:** Set goals that fit your lifestyle—if you're new to exercise, walking three days a week is more realistic than daily marathon training.
- **Relevant:** Target behaviors directly linked to blood sugar control, like meal planning or regular activity.
- **Time-bound:** Set a timeframe, such as "for the next four weeks," to create urgency and focus.

What began as a manageable commitment soon blossomed into a daily ritual. With each milestone—walking five days a week, then incorporating weekend hikes—Maya saw her blood sugar levels stabilize and her energy soar. Over time, these small victories accumulated, leading to reduced medication and a profound sense of self-efficacy. Maya's story is a testament to the fact that sustainable change is built on practical, personalized goals.

Cultural Perspectives: Goal-Setting Across the Globe

Goal-setting is a universal tool, but its expression can be shaped by culture. In Japan, for instance, the concept of **kaizen**—continuous, incremental improvement—has been applied to health behaviors with great success. Rather than dramatic overhauls, individuals focus on making one small positive change each day, such as swapping white rice for brown or practicing mindful breathing before meals.

Meanwhile, in Scandinavian countries, community-based programs encourage group goal-setting, where peers provide support and accountability. This collective approach has led to notable improvements in diabetes outcomes, highlighting the value of shared goals and social connection.

Your Goal-Setting Blueprint

To set effective goals for your own journey, consider the following process:

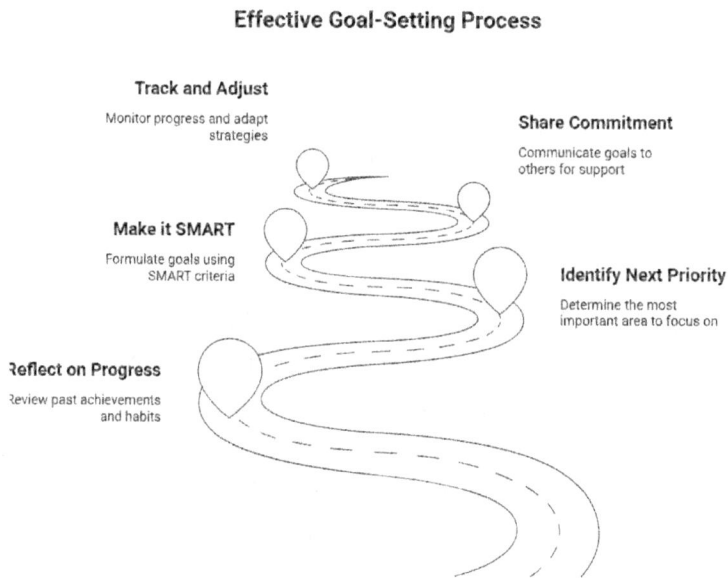

Effective Goal-Setting Process

Track and Adjust
Monitor progress and adapt strategies

Share Commitment
Communicate goals to others for support

Make it SMART
Formulate goals using SMART criteria

Identify Next Priority
Determine the most important area to focus on

Reflect on Progress
Review past achievements and habits

- **Reflect on your progress:** What habits have you already changed? What's working?
- **Identify your next priority:** Is it nutrition, movement, stress, or sleep?
- **Make it SMART:** Write your goal using the five SMART criteria.
- **Share your commitment:** Tell a friend, family member, or your healthcare provider.

- **Track and adjust:** Regularly review your progress and adapt as needed.

Examples of positive goals:

- "I will prepare a plant-based lunch three times a week."
- "I will practice deep breathing for five minutes before bed each night."
- "I will check my blood sugar after breakfast and record the results for one month."

Overcoming Setbacks and Celebrating Success

No journey is linear. There will be days when motivation wanes or unexpected obstacles arise. The key is to view setbacks as learning opportunities, not failures. When you achieve a goal, celebrate—no matter how small the milestone. Rewards reinforce positive behavior and remind you of your capacity for change.

```
- Consistently setting and tracking realistic goals can reduce HbA1c levels by
up to 1-2% within six months, a clinically significant improvement for type 2
diabetes management.
- Studies show that individuals who engage in goal-oriented self-management
have a lower risk of diabetes-related complications over the long term.
```

Setting new goals is the linchpin between your past achievements and your future health. By crafting meaningful, personalized objectives, you empower yourself to continue the journey toward lasting wellness. In the next section, we'll explore how to maintain your momentum and prevent relapse, ensuring that your new beginning becomes a lifelong transformation.

14.3 Staying Connected

Human transformation rarely happens in isolation. While your efforts to reverse type 2 diabetes have been grounded in personal commitment and daily choices, the path to lasting health becomes more sustainable—and rewarding—when you stay connected. This final phase is not just about continuing what you've started, but about weaving your new life into a supportive network, drawing strength from others, and offering inspiration in return.

The Power of Community

Isolation is a risk factor for relapse. Studies have shown that people who remain engaged with family, friends, healthcare professionals, and peer groups are significantly more likely to maintain positive health changes. This is especially true in managing chronic conditions like type 2 diabetes, where accountability, encouragement, and collective wisdom can make the difference between temporary improvement and lifelong success.

The Role of Community in Health Management

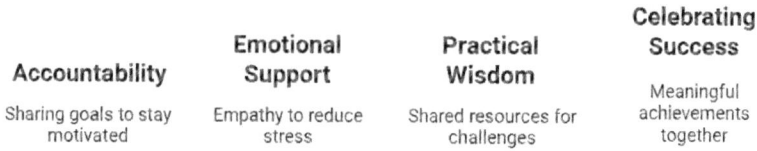

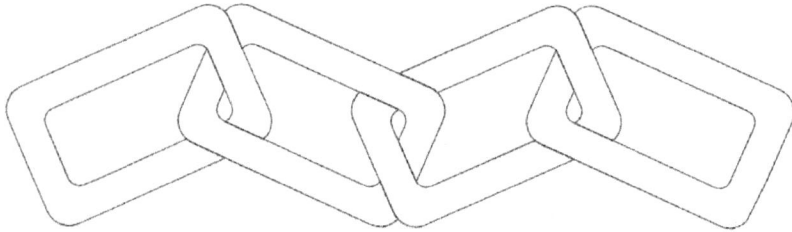

Accountability	Emotional Support	Practical Wisdom	Celebrating Success
Sharing goals to stay motivated	Empathy to reduce stress	Shared resources for challenges	Meaningful achievements together

- **Accountability:** Sharing your goals and progress with others helps keep you motivated.

- **Emotional Support:** Managing diabetes can be challenging. Empathy from those who understand your journey can mitigate stress and emotional fatigue.

- **Practical Wisdom:** Groups offer shared resources, tips, and solutions for daily challenges.

- **Celebrating Success:** Achievements—large or small—feel more meaningful when celebrated together.

Real-World Example: The Village Model

In Japan, where community living and group activities are deeply ingrained, diabetes support groups have shown remarkable effectiveness. In the rural town of Minamiuonuma, local health authorities established "health circles" where residents meet weekly to cook healthy meals, exercise, and discuss their progress. Over five years, participants experienced significant reductions in blood sugar levels and medication dependence. The secret wasn't just diet or exercise—it was the power of shared commitment and mutual encouragement.

Staying Connected Digitally

Not everyone has access to local support groups, but technology bridges the gap. Online communities, forums, and social media groups devoted to diabetes management provide a sense of belonging and immediate access to guidance. Apps can connect you to health coaches, track your progress, and even alert your care team to changes in your condition.

> Diabetes-focused forums (such as **Diabetes Daily** or **TuDiabetes**)
> Social media support groups (Facebook, WhatsApp, local platforms)
> Telemedicine programs for regular check-ins with healthcare providers

Building Your Personal Support Network

- **Identify Key Allies:** Family members, close friends, and trusted healthcare professionals.
- **Communicate Your Goals:** Let your network know what you're working toward and how they can help.
- **Set Up Regular Check-Ins:** Weekly or monthly conversations to share progress and setbacks.
- **Join or Start a Group:** Whether local or virtual, a group keeps you inspired and accountable.

Personal Story: Rajiv's Journey

Rajiv, a 54-year-old engineer from Mumbai, struggled with type 2 diabetes for over a decade. After years of fluctuating blood sugar levels and multiple medications, he made a commitment to change. However, it wasn't until his wife joined him in morning walks and his colleagues created a lunchtime walking club that Rajiv truly found momentum. "We encouraged each other, shared recipes, even celebrated milestones together," Rajiv recalls. "I felt like I wasn't alone. That made all the difference." A year later, Rajiv's doctor reduced his medications, and his A1C levels stabilized. For Rajiv, connection was the catalyst for transformation.

Cultural Perspectives on Connectedness

Different cultures offer unique approaches to staying connected. In many Indigenous communities, health is viewed as a collective responsibility, with elders, family, and community leaders playing active roles in supporting individuals with chronic illnesses. In Scandinavian countries, social clubs and communal activities are integral to maintaining health and well-being, offering models for how shared experiences can lead to better outcomes.

Tips for Maintaining Connection

> Be proactive: Don't wait for others to reach out—initiate contact.
> Practice vulnerability: Share both your triumphs and struggles honestly.
> Give back: Supporting others in their journey can reinforce your commitment.

Celebrate together: Mark your progress with shared meals, outings, or virtual hangouts.

The Lifelong Benefits

Maintaining these connections doesn't just help you manage diabetes—it enriches your life in countless ways. Social ties have been linked to lower rates of depression, improved heart health, and even longer lifespan. Most importantly, staying connected turns your journey from a solitary struggle into a shared celebration.

```
People with strong social support networks are up to 50% more likely to
achieve long-term remission of type 2 diabetes.
Regular participation in community or peer support groups can reduce diabetes-
related stress and improve blood sugar control.
```

Cultivating a supportive community is your anchor for sustainable change. Whether it's a walking group, a digital forum, or simply a trusted friend, these connections will help you weather setbacks and amplify your successes. As you move forward, remember that your story can also inspire others. In the next section, we'll discuss how to keep your momentum going and protect your progress, ensuring that your new beginning continues to blossom into lasting health.

14.4 The Power of Advocacy

The journey to reversing type 2 diabetes is rarely a solitary path. As you've discovered, the habits you form and the knowledge you gain not only transform your own life but can also spark change in those around you. **Advocacy**—the act of championing a cause, sharing your story, and supporting others—can be a powerful force in sustaining your newfound health and inspiring others to begin their own journeys.

When you advocate for yourself, you become an active participant in your health care. No longer a passive recipient of advice, you ask questions, seek resources, and ensure your voice is heard. This proactive stance often leads to better outcomes, deeper understanding, and the confidence to make informed choices about your well-being.

The Ripple Effect: Inspiring Change Beyond Yourself

Personal advocacy doesn't end with self-care. By sharing your experiences—whether it's your initial diagnosis, your struggles and triumphs with dietary changes, or the moment you first saw your blood sugar drop into healthy ranges—you create a ripple effect. Others see what's possible and are encouraged to believe in their own potential for change.

Consider the story of **Amina**, a teacher from Nairobi, Kenya. Diagnosed with type 2 diabetes in her late forties, she initially felt isolated and overwhelmed. After learning about the importance of whole grains, local leafy greens, and regular walking,

Amina not only reversed her own insulin resistance but also started a weekly health group at her school. Her advocacy led to the school canteen introducing lower-glycemic index options, benefiting both staff and students. Amina's journey illustrates how one person's commitment can transform a community.

Advocacy in Action: Practical Steps

Advocacy can take many forms, from everyday conversations to organized community initiatives. Here are some practical ways you can become an advocate for lasting health:

- **Share your story**: Talk openly about your diagnosis, lifestyle changes, and successes. Authentic stories resonate and inspire.
- **Educate your circle**: Offer to share what you've learned about glycemic index, meal planning, or stress reduction with family, friends, or colleagues.
- **Support others**: Volunteer at local diabetes support groups, participate in online forums, or mentor someone newly diagnosed.
- **Partner with healthcare professionals**: Work with your doctor or dietitian to develop accessible educational materials, or provide feedback on how patient care can improve.
- **Influence policy and environment**: Advocate for healthier food options in schools, workplaces, or community centers. This might mean petitioning for fresh produce in local stores or organizing walking clubs.

Historical Perspective: Advocacy's Lasting Impact

History is rich with examples of advocacy changing the course of health and disease. In the early 20th century, **Dr. Elliott Joslin**, an American physician, was among the first to champion patient self-management in diabetes care. At a time when few believed that diet and exercise could alter disease outcomes, Joslin's tireless advocacy led to the development of patient education programs and the first diabetes self-management clinics in Boston. His work has had a lasting influence, shaping modern diabetes care worldwide.

Similarly, in India, the **Diabetes Foundation** was established by healthcare professionals and patient advocates in the late 1970s. This organization promoted public awareness, early screening, and community-based interventions long before diabetes became a national epidemic. Their advocacy efforts helped shift public perception, reduce stigma, and bring diabetes management into the mainstream.

A Timeline of Advocacy: From Personal to Global

- **Personal Commitment**: You choose to take control of your health, learn about diabetes, and make daily changes.
- **Sharing Your Story**: You open up to friends and family, breaking down barriers and myths.
- **Community Engagement**: You join or create local groups, expand your reach, and empower others.
- **Systemic Change**: Collectively, advocates push for healthier environments, better policies, and improved healthcare services.

The momentum created through individual and collective advocacy can lead to societal shifts—making healthy choices the norm rather than the exception.

Building a Network: The Power of Collective Advocacy

Connecting with others who share your goals magnifies your impact. Diverse perspectives—whether from different cultural backgrounds, age groups, or regions—enrich the conversation and broaden the movement. For example, a group of friends in Mexico City, inspired by one member's reversal of type 2 diabetes, started a neighborhood initiative to promote traditional, lower-glycemic Mexican dishes at local markets. Their advocacy not only improved their own health but also reinforced cultural heritage.

Very important: Research shows that peer support and community advocacy significantly improve diabetes self-management, leading to better long-term health outcomes.

Advocacy is more than a buzzword—it's a lifeline, a way to sustain your progress and help others unlock their potential for lasting health. Whether you share your story with one person or champion systemic change, your efforts matter. In the next section, we'll explore how to safeguard your progress, maintain your momentum, and continue building a life defined by vitality and hope. Your new beginning isn't just about your own future; it's about lighting the way for others to follow.

14.5 Your Next Steps

As you stand at the threshold of this new beginning, the path toward lasting health is illuminated by the choices you make—one step at a time. Lasting change is rarely the result of a single decision, but rather a series of intentional actions, each reinforcing your resolve and shaping your future. Now is the moment to translate knowledge into action, transforming the insights and strategies explored throughout this book into daily practice.

Take a moment to reflect on your personal motivations. Are you driven by the desire to reclaim energy, reduce reliance on medication, or be present for loved ones? By clarifying your "why," you anchor your journey in meaning, empowering yourself to persevere through challenges.

Mapping Out Your Personalized Plan

A successful health journey is not a rigid script but a flexible roadmap—one that adapts to your unique lifestyle, culture, and preferences. Here's how you can chart your course:

- **Define Measurable Goals**

  - Set specific, realistic objectives (e.g., lowering your A1C by a certain percentage, walking 30 minutes daily, or preparing more home-cooked meals).
  - Use a journal or app to track your progress and celebrate milestones.

- **Establish Support Systems**

  - Enlist the support of family, friends, or a healthcare provider.
  - Join a diabetes support group, either locally or online, to share experiences and advice.

- **Create a Sustainable Routine**

  - Build routines around meals, exercise, and self-care that fit your daily life.
  - Schedule regular check-ins to reassess your goals and adapt as needed.

- **Prepare for Setbacks**

  - Anticipate that obstacles may arise and plan for how you'll respond.

  - Practice self-compassion—remember, progress is not always linear.

Real-World Inspirations

Let's pause to highlight the journeys of others who have walked this path before you.

Consider **Anita's story** from Mumbai, India. Diagnosed with type 2 diabetes at age 52, Anita initially felt overwhelmed by the dietary restrictions and medication regimen. With guidance from her doctor, she embraced a plant-based diet rich in lentils, vegetables, and traditional spices. She began walking with her neighbors each morning, transforming exercise into a social ritual. Over 18 months, Anita not only reduced her blood sugar levels and medication but also inspired friends and family to adopt healthier habits.

Half a world away, in the United States, **Carlos** faced a different set of challenges. As a father of three, working two jobs, he found it difficult to prioritize his health. After attending a community workshop on diabetes management, Carlos started making small changes: swapping sugary drinks for water, choosing brown rice over white, and involving his children in preparing healthy meals. These incremental shifts added up, and within a year, Carlos saw significant improvements in his A1C levels and energy.

These stories reflect a universal truth—lasting health is attainable, regardless of background or circumstance, when you commit to actionable steps and seek support.

Action Steps for the Next 30 Days

To help you maintain momentum, here's a simple 30-day action plan:

- **Week 1: Build Awareness**

  - Track your meals and blood sugar responses.
  - Identify high and low glycemic foods in your diet.

- **Week 2: Make One Change**

  - Choose one meal to optimize (e.g., swap white bread for whole grains).
  - Add 10 minutes of physical activity to your day.

- **Week 3: Expand Your Toolbox**

  - Try a new stress-reduction technique (deep breathing, meditation, or yoga).
  - Connect with a support group or accountability partner.

- **Week 4: Reflect and Adjust**

  - Review your progress, noting successes and challenges.
  - Set new goals for the month ahead.

Building a Foundation for the Future

Remember, reversing type 2 diabetes is often a process of sustained transformation rather than a quick fix. Each new habit, every supportive conversation, and all the mindful choices you make contribute to a foundation of lasting health. You are not alone—millions around the world are on a similar journey, sharing triumphs and setbacks, learning and growing together.

Essential Facts to Carry Forward

- Even modest weight loss (5-10% of body weight) can significantly improve blood sugar control and reduce diabetes complications.

```
- Consistently choosing low glycemic index foods helps stabilize blood glucose
and can lower the risk of long-term complications.
```

Moving Forward Together

Your next steps signal more than personal progress—they offer hope to your community and future generations. By embodying resilience, compassion, and determination, you become a beacon for others facing similar challenges. As you continue to refine your habits and routines, remember that every positive choice, no matter how small, is a victory worth celebrating.

In summary, your journey toward reversing type 2 diabetes is a testament to the power of informed action and sustained commitment. As you move forward, embrace each day as a fresh opportunity to nurture your health and inspire those around you.

14.6 Closing Thoughts

As you arrive at this pivotal point in your journey toward reversing type 2 diabetes, it's important to pause and reflect on the path you've traveled so far. The road to lasting health is not a sprint, but a purposeful walk—each step informed by knowledge, guided by evidence, and empowered by your own determination. Throughout this book, you've encountered scientific explanations, practical strategies, and inspiring stories, all woven together to illuminate the real possibility of reclaiming your health.

Embracing Change: The Power of Small Steps

Change often feels daunting, especially when it involves deeply ingrained habits around food, activity, and self-care. Yet, as we've seen, true transformation is not about overnight miracles, but about consistent, incremental progress. Consider the story of **Manuel**, a retiree from Mexico City. Diagnosed with type 2 diabetes in his early 60s, Manuel was overwhelmed by the dietary restrictions and medication schedules suddenly thrust upon him. Initially, he tried drastic diets that left him frustrated and fatigued. It wasn't until he focused on small, sustainable changes—swapping white rice for whole grains, taking evening walks with his granddaughter, and learning to prepare traditional dishes with fresh vegetables—that he began to see a meaningful shift. Over a year, not only did Manuel lower his A1C, but he also rekindled a sense of joy in daily life.

His story echoes the experience of **Priya**, a schoolteacher in India. Her family's meals were rich in starchy staples, and she struggled to balance her blood sugar despite her best intentions. With the support of a local diabetes education group, Priya discovered the power of the **glycemic index** and learned how to blend lentils, leafy greens, and low-GI grains into her meals. By making these culturally resonant adaptations, Priya achieved better glucose control and became an advocate for healthy eating in her community.

These real-world examples demonstrate that while the underlying science of diabetes management is universal, the path to health can—and should—be tailored to your unique culture, preferences, and resources.

Key Takeaways for Lifelong Success

As you look ahead, remember that the journey to lasting health is sustained by a few core principles:

Knowledge is power: Understanding the science of type 2 diabetes empowers you to make informed choices every day.

Flexibility matters: Adapt dietary and lifestyle strategies to your culture, taste, and personal circumstances.

Support is essential: Surround yourself with a network—be it family, friends, or a community group—who understands and encourages your goals.

Consistency outweighs perfection: Sustainable change is about what you do most of the time, not about never making a mistake.

Practical Timeline: Your Ongoing Journey

- **First Month**: Focus on understanding your baseline—track your blood sugar, meals, and activity.
- **Months 2-3**: Implement gradual changes—adjust your diet, try new recipes, and establish a regular exercise pattern.
- **Months 4-6**: Monitor your progress, celebrate small victories, and seek support if you encounter setbacks.
- **Beyond 6 Months**: Continue building on your successes, revisit your goals, and remain open to learning and adapting.

The Global Perspective: A Shared Challenge

Type 2 diabetes is a global epidemic, affecting people across continents and cultures. Yet, as we've explored, the solutions are often rooted in local traditions—Mediterranean diets rich in olive oil and legumes, East Asian meals centered around vegetables and fermented foods, or African dishes featuring whole grains and pulses. By learning from diverse approaches, we broaden our toolkit for managing and reversing diabetes, and we honor the wisdom embedded in global food cultures.

The Science of Hope

Perhaps the most important lesson is that diabetes is not a life sentence. For decades, the prevailing narrative was one of inevitable decline—progressively higher blood sugars, more medications, and mounting complications. Recent research, however, has rewritten that story. We now know that with dedicated lifestyle changes, many people can achieve remission, reduce medication dependency, and restore their quality of life.

Fact: Studies show that up to 60% of people with type 2 diabetes can achieve remission through sustained weight loss, dietary change, and increased physical activity.

Very Important: The earlier you begin making changes, the greater your chances of reversing the course of type 2 diabetes and preventing complications.

Moving Forward: Your New Beginning

As you close this chapter, remember that your journey is uniquely your own. There will be challenges, setbacks, and unexpected victories. If you ever feel discouraged, recall the stories of Manuel and Priya, and the countless others who have walked this path before you. Let their resilience inspire your next step.

Above all, embrace the journey as a new beginning—a chance not only to manage a medical condition, but to reclaim your vitality, deepen your sense of well-being, and connect more fully with the world around you.

In summary, reversing type 2 diabetes is both a personal and communal journey, rooted in knowledge and sustained by hope. As you continue, turn to the next chapter for practical resources and tools that will help you put these lessons into action, ensuring your path to lasting health remains clear, achievable, and deeply rewarding.

Glossary

A1C (Hemoglobin A1C)

A1C is a blood test that measures the average level of blood sugar (glucose) over the past two to three months. It is expressed as a percentage. Higher A1C values indicate poorer blood sugar control and increased risk of diabetes complications. Regular monitoring helps assess the effectiveness of diabetes management strategies.

Beta Cells

Beta cells are specialized cells in the pancreas responsible for producing and releasing insulin, the hormone that regulates blood glucose levels. In type 2 diabetes, beta cells may become dysfunctional or die due to chronic high blood sugar, inflammation, or stress. Preserving beta cell health is crucial to reversing diabetes.

Blood Glucose

Blood glucose refers to the amount of sugar present in the bloodstream. This level rises after eating and falls as the body uses or stores glucose. Chronically high blood glucose is a hallmark of diabetes and can lead to serious health complications if not managed effectively.

Carbohydrates

Carbohydrates are one of the three main macronutrients found in foods, alongside protein and fat. They are the body's primary source of energy, but they directly impact blood sugar levels. Managing carbohydrate intake—especially the type and amount—is essential for diabetes control.

Complex Carbohydrates

Complex carbohydrates are long chains of sugar molecules found in foods like whole grains, legumes, and vegetables. They are digested more slowly than simple carbohydrates, causing a gradual rise in blood sugar. Including complex carbs in a diabetes-friendly diet helps with blood sugar stability.

Continuous Glucose Monitor (CGM)

A CGM is a wearable device that tracks blood glucose levels in real-time, providing continuous feedback. It helps individuals see the immediate effects of food, exercise, and lifestyle choices on their glucose levels, enabling more precise diabetes management.

Diabetes Remission

Diabetes remission refers to achieving and maintaining normal blood sugar levels without the need for diabetes medications. This state is often reached through lifestyle changes such as diet, exercise, and weight loss. Remission is different from a cure, as relapse can occur if old habits return

Diabetic Neuropathy

Diabetic neuropathy is nerve damage caused by high blood sugar in people with diabetes. It commonly affects the feet and hands, leading to numbness, pain, or weakness. Preventing or managing neuropathy involves maintaining good blood sugar control and adopting healthy lifestyle habits.

Dietary Fiber

Dietary fiber is the indigestible part of plant-based foods that helps regulate digestion and blood sugar. Foods high in fiber, such as vegetables, fruits, and whole grains, slow glucose absorption and improve insulin sensitivity, making them essential for diabetes management.

Glycemic Index (GI)

The glycemic index is a ranking system for carbohydrates based on how quickly they raise blood sugar levels after consumption. Foods with a high GI cause rapid spikes, while low-GI foods result in gradual increases. Managing GI in food choices is key for blood sugar control.

Glycemic Load (GL)

Glycemic load considers both the glycemic index and the amount of carbohydrate in a serving of food. It provides a more comprehensive picture of a food's impact on blood sugar. Lower GL foods are preferred for diabetes management.

Hyperglycemia

Hyperglycemia refers to abnormally high blood glucose levels. It can result from overeating, inadequate insulin, illness, or stress. Persistent hyperglycemia can lead to serious complications, making prompt management essential.

Hypoglycemia

Hypoglycemia is a condition of abnormally low blood glucose levels, often caused by excessive insulin or missed meals. Symptoms include shakiness, confusion, and fainting. Managing medication and food intake helps prevent hypoglycemia in people with diabetes.

Insulin

Insulin is a hormone produced by the pancreas that allows cells to absorb glucose from the blood for energy. In type 2 diabetes, the body either resists insulin's effects or does not produce enough. Strategies that improve insulin sensitivity are key to reversing diabetes.

Insulin Resistance

Insulin resistance occurs when the body's cells do not respond properly to insulin, forcing the pancreas to produce more and leading to elevated blood glucose. This is a central feature of type 2 diabetes and can be improved through exercise and dietary changes.

Lifestyle Modification

Lifestyle modification refers to changes in daily habits—such as diet, physical activity, sleep, and stress management—that support health and disease prevention. For type 2 diabetes, these changes are often the most effective way to achieve remission or significant improvement.

Mediterranean Diet

The Mediterranean diet is a plant-forward eating pattern rich in vegetables, fruits, whole grains, legumes, nuts, olive oil, and lean proteins. Research shows it can improve blood glucose control and reduce cardiovascular risk, making it a popular choice for diabetes management.

Metabolic Syndrome

Metabolic syndrome is a cluster of conditions—including high blood pressure, high blood sugar, excess abdominal fat, and abnormal cholesterol—that increase the risk of type 2 diabetes and heart disease. Early intervention can prevent progression to full-blown diabetes.

Microvascular Complications

Microvascular complications are diabetes-related damages to small blood vessels, affecting organs like the eyes (retinopathy), kidneys (nephropathy), and nerves (neuropathy). Preventing these complications requires consistent blood sugar control and healthy lifestyle choices

Non-Insulin Medications

These are oral or injectable medications used to lower blood sugar in people with type 2 diabetes who do not require insulin. Examples include metformin, GLP-1 agonists, and SGLT2 inhibitors. Lifestyle changes can sometimes reduce or eliminate the need for these drugs.

Oral Glucose Tolerance Test (OGTT)

The OGTT is a diagnostic test that measures the body's ability to manage a glucose load. After fasting, the patient consumes a sugary drink, and blood glucose is measured at intervals. It helps diagnose diabetes and prediabetes.

Pancreas

The pancreas is an organ located behind the stomach, responsible for producing insulin and digestive enzymes. In type 2 diabetes, the pancreas may struggle to compensate for insulin resistance, leading to elevated blood sugar.

Plant-Based Diet

A plant-based diet emphasizes vegetables, fruits, whole grains, legumes, nuts, and seeds, and limits animal products. This approach is associated with improved insulin sensitivity and lower risk of type 2 diabetes. Variations exist globally, such as vegetarian and vegan diets.

Prediabetes

Prediabetes is a condition where blood glucose levels are higher than normal but not high enough to be classified as diabetes. It is a warning sign and can often be reversed with lifestyle changes, preventing progression to type 2 diabetes.

Reverse (Reversal of Diabetes)

Reversal of diabetes means achieving normal blood sugar levels without medication, typically through sustained lifestyle changes. It does not imply a cure, as relapse can occur if healthy habits are not maintained.

Self-Monitoring of Blood Glucose (SMBG)

SMBG involves regularly checking blood sugar levels at home using a glucometer. This practice empowers individuals to understand their response to food, exercise, and stress, and to adjust their routines accordingly.

Simple Carbohydrates

Simple carbohydrates are sugars or products containing refined grains that are quickly digested, causing rapid increases in blood sugar. Sources include table sugar, candy, white bread, and sweetened beverages. Limiting these is important for diabetes control.

Stress Management

Stress management includes practices—such as mindfulness, yoga, deep breathing, or cultural rituals—that help reduce psychological stress. Chronic stress can worsen blood sugar control, while effective management supports diabetes reversal.

Type 2 Diabetes

Type 2 diabetes is a chronic condition characterized by high blood sugar due to insulin resistance and impaired insulin production. It is influenced by genetics, lifestyle, and environment. Unlike type 1 diabetes, it can often be managed or reversed through lifestyle changes.

Vegetarian Diet

A vegetarian diet excludes meat but may include dairy and eggs. It can support diabetes management if well-designed, emphasizing whole foods, fiber, and balanced nutrients. Cultural variations influence specific vegetarian practices worldwide.

This glossary provides a foundational understanding of essential terms related to reversing type 2 diabetes. These definitions offer context, linkages, and examples to foster deeper comprehension as you explore strategies for lasting health. Each term connects to broader themes of lifestyle change, global diversity, and the science underpinning diabetes management.

Annexure A: The Evolution of Diabetes Understanding

This annexure provides readers with a sweeping historical perspective on how type 2 diabetes has been understood, diagnosed, and treated across centuries. By tracing the shifting landscape of diabetes knowledge and interventions, it connects the present-day approach to the lessons, successes, and failures of the past, illuminating how cultural, scientific, and medical paradigms have shaped current strategies in reversing type 2 diabetes.

The Timeline of Diabetes Understanding and Management

1. Ancient Beginnings

1550 BCE – The Ebers Papyrus: The earliest known reference to diabetes symptoms appears in ancient Egypt, where excessive urination is noted. The condition, then unnamed, was mystifying to physicians.

5th–6th Century CE – India and the Honey Urine Test: Indian physicians reference "Madhumeha" (honey urine), observing that ants are attracted to the sweet urine of affected individuals, an early recognition of diabetes.

2. Classical and Medieval Observations

2nd Century CE – Aretaeus of Cappadocia: A Greek physician formally names the disease "diabetes," derived from the Greek "siphon," describing the passing of water through the body.

10th–11th Century CE – Avicenna's Canon of Medicine: The Persian polymath Avicenna describes diabetes in detail, noting complications such as gangrene. His work underscores the disease's growing recognition in the Islamic Golden Age.

3. The Age of Scientific Discovery

18th Century – Thomas Willis: An English physician identifies the sweet taste of diabetic urine, leading to the term "diabetes mellitus" ("mellitus" meaning honey-sweet).

19th Century – Claude Bernard: French physiologist Bernard discovers the role of the liver in glucose production, hinting at the metabolic roots of diabetes.

4. Insulin and Beyond

1921 – Insulin's Discovery: Frederick Banting and Charles Best at the University of Toronto isolate insulin, transforming diabetes management from fatal to manageable. Before this, dietary starvation was the only recourse for survival.

1950s–1970s – Oral Medications Emerge: The development of sulfonylureas and biguanides allows for non-insulin therapies, marking the dawn of modern pharmaceutical interventions.

5. Modern Paradigms: Lifestyle and Prevention

1980s–2000s – The Global Diabetes Epidemic: Rising rates of type 2 diabetes prompt the World Health Organization and the International Diabetes Federation to declare a global crisis, shifting focus to prevention and lifestyle change.

2010s–Present – Remission and Reversal: Groundbreaking studies demonstrate that significant weight loss, diet modification, and increased physical activity can induce remission in type 2 diabetes, ushering in a new era of hope and empowerment.

Examples and Applications

Example 1: Banting's Breakthrough and Its Legacy

Frederick Banting's relentless pursuit of a treatment for diabetes in the early 20th century not only resulted in the first therapeutic use of insulin but also galvanized global research into metabolic diseases. His story demonstrates the impact of scientific curiosity and perseverance—qualities that continue to drive innovation in diabetes reversal strategies today.

Example 2: The Newcastle Remission Study

In the 2010s, researchers at Newcastle University in the UK conducted landmark studies proving that intensive dietary intervention could reverse type 2 diabetes in many individuals. Participants followed a very low-calorie diet and, within weeks, experienced normalized blood sugar levels. This modern application echoes historical dietary approaches but with the benefit of scientific rigor, proving that the roots of reversal are often found in the past.

This historical journey underscores that our understanding of type 2 diabetes has evolved dramatically—from fatalistic resignation to hopeful reversal. By appreciating these milestones, readers can contextualize today's recommendations and recognize that every step forward stands on the shoulders of centuries of inquiry and adaptation.

Annexure B: Global Perspectives—Cultural Practices

This annexure delves into the rich tapestry of cultural responses to diabetes around the world. By exploring dietary traditions, community health models, and culturally-specific interventions, it highlights how understanding and reversing type 2 diabetes is a universal challenge approached in diverse ways. This global lens reinforces the book's core message: sustainable health strategies must respect and integrate cultural context.

Cultural Approaches to Diabetes Management

1. The Mediterranean Diet—A Model of Prevention and Reversal

Origins and Principles: Rooted in the traditional eating patterns of Greece, Italy, and neighboring regions, the Mediterranean diet emphasizes whole grains, legumes, vegetables, olive oil, moderate fish, and minimal processed foods.

Scientific Backing: Numerous studies, including the PREDIMED trial in Spain, have demonstrated that this dietary pattern reduces the risk of developing type 2 diabetes and supports glycemic control in those already diagnosed.

2. India's Plant-Based Heritage and Modern Challenges

Vegetarian Traditions: Vegetarianism in India, practiced for religious and ethical reasons, naturally emphasizes legumes, whole grains, and vegetables. Historically, these diets have been associated with lower diabetes prevalence.

Urbanization and Processed Foods: Recent shifts toward highly processed foods and sedentary lifestyles have led to a surge in type 2 diabetes, particularly in urban centers. However, a return to traditional plant-based meals is now championed by public health advocates.

3. Indigenous Wisdom—The Pima People of North America

Traditional Diets: The Pima, indigenous to the southwestern United States and northern Mexico, once thrived on a diet of beans, squash, corn, and wild foods, with virtually no diabetes.

Lifestyle Disruption: The introduction of processed foods and reduced physical activity in the 20th century led to skyrocketing diabetes rates. Community-led programs are now seeking to revive traditional eating and activity patterns, resulting in improved health outcomes.

Examples and Applications

Example 1: The Blue Zones Phenomenon

Epidemiologist Dan Buettner identified "Blue Zones"—regions where people live exceptionally long, healthy lives. Among them, the Greek island of Ikaria and Okinawa, Japan, have notably low rates of type 2 diabetes. Their secret: plant-heavy diets, regular movement, strong social networks, and minimal processed food. These cultural artifacts provide living proof that lifestyle is powerful medicine.

Example 2: Maori Community Initiatives in New Zealand

The Maori population has experienced high rates of type 2 diabetes following the colonization and dietary shifts. Community-led programs that revive traditional food cultivation (kumara, taro, native greens) and promote group exercise are showing promise in reducing diabetes prevalence. These efforts underline the importance of cultural identity in health restoration.

This global journey reveals that the roots of diabetes reversal are often found in cultural wisdom and community resilience. Strategies that honor local traditions, foodways, and social structures are not only more respectful but also more effective. Readers are encouraged to see their health journey as part of a broader tapestry—one where culture, community, and science meet.

Annexure C: Key Scientific Studies—Primary Source Insights

This annexure presents excerpts and summaries from landmark scientific studies that have shaped our current understanding of type 2 diabetes reversal. By offering a window into the evidence base, it empowers readers to appreciate the rigor underpinning the book's recommendations and demystifies the science behind sustainable change.

Pivotal Research Summaries and Excerpts

1. The DiRECT Trial—Remission Through Diet

Study Summary: The Diabetes Remission Clinical Trial (DiRECT), published in 2017 in the UK, assessed whether a structured, low-calorie diet could induce remission in people with type 2 diabetes.

Key Findings: Nearly half (46%) of participants achieved remission at 12 months, defined as normal blood sugar levels without medication.

Excerpt: "Our data show that remission of type 2 diabetes is achievable for many people, with major implications for health systems worldwide." — Dr. Roy Taylor, DiRECT Principal Investigator

2. Look AHEAD—The Power of Lifestyle Change

Study Summary: The Look AHEAD (Action for Health in Diabetes) study followed over 5,000 overweight or obese adults with type 2 diabetes in the US, testing the impact of intensive lifestyle intervention.

Key Findings: Participants lost more weight, improved fitness, and had better glycemic control than those receiving standard care.

Excerpt: "Intensive lifestyle intervention produces greater weight loss and improvements in fitness and glycemic control than standard support and education." — The Look AHEAD Research Group

3. The Finnish Diabetes Prevention Study (DPS)

Study Summary: This landmark trial demonstrated that people at high risk for type 2 diabetes could prevent or delay its onset through weight loss, dietary changes, and increased activity.

Key Findings: Incidence of diabetes was reduced by 58% among those receiving the lifestyle intervention.

Excerpt: "Sustained changes in lifestyle can substantially reduce the risk of type 2 diabetes in high-risk individuals." — Tuomilehto et al., New England Journal of Medicine, 2001

Examples and Applications

Example 1: Translating Research to Daily Life

The DiRECT trial's focus on meal replacement shakes and calorie restriction may not suit everyone, but its underlying principle—significant, sustained dietary change—can be adapted culturally. For example, in Japan, "shokuiku" (food education) programs teach balanced, portion-controlled meals rooted in tradition, echoing the trial's approach in a local context.

Example 2: Community-Based Lifestyle Programs

The Finnish DPS inspired similar interventions worldwide, such as the US Diabetes Prevention Program (DPP) and India's D-CLIP trial. These initiatives have demonstrated that group-based support, regular check-ins, and culturally tailored advice make a measurable difference in diabetes prevention and reversal.

Scientific breakthroughs are not distant abstractions but practical guides for real people. By grounding lifestyle change in robust evidence, readers can trust that their efforts are not only hopeful but also proven. This annexure bridges the gap between the laboratory and everyday life, reinforcing the book's evidence-based path to lasting health.

Annexure D: Glycemic Index and Glycemic Load

This annexure serves as a user-friendly resource for understanding and applying the concepts of **glycemic index (GI)** and **glycemic load (GL)** in daily life. By breaking down these tools and providing real-world food examples, it helps readers make informed choices to optimize blood sugar control and support diabetes reversal.

Understanding GI and GL

What is the Glycemic Index?

Definition: GI measures how quickly a carbohydrate-containing food raises blood glucose levels compared to pure glucose (GI = 100).

Categories:

- Low GI: 55 or less

- Medium GI: 56–69

- High GI: 70 or more

What is Glycemic Load?

Definition: GL takes into account both the GI and the amount of carbohydrate in a typical serving, providing a more accurate reflection of a food's real-world impact on blood sugar.

Calculation: GL = (GI x grams of carbohydrate per serving) / 100

Categories:

- Low GL: 10 or less

- Medium GL: 11–19

- High GL: 20 or more

Practical Food Examples

Low GI and Low GL Foods

Lentils (GI: 32, GL: 5 per serving): A staple in many cultures, lentils are filling, nutritious, and gentle on blood sugar.

Non-starchy vegetables (GI: varies, GL: very low): Broccoli, spinach, and peppers are excellent daily choices.

Barley (GI: 28, GL: 9): Used in soups and salads worldwide, barley is both hearty and diabetes-friendly.

High GI and High GL Foods

White bread (GI: 75, GL: 15 per slice): Common in Western diets but best minimized.

Instant rice (GI: 85, GL: 17 per serving): Often used for convenience, but traditional brown rice is a much better option.

Potato chips (GI: 70, GL: 12 per serving): Widely consumed snack with a high impact on blood sugar.

Application: Building a Balanced Plate

Start with Low GI Carbohydrates: Choose whole grains, legumes, and non-starchy vegetables as your meal's foundation.

Add Lean Protein: Protein helps slow carbohydrate absorption.

Include Healthy Fats: Olive oil, nuts, and avocado add satiety and further reduce the meal's glycemic impact.

Limit High GI Foods: Reserve them for occasional treats and pair them with fiber and protein to blunt blood sugar spikes.

Example: A Day of Low GI/GL Meals

Breakfast: Oatmeal (GI: 55, GL: 13) with berries and a handful of walnuts

Lunch: Lentil soup, mixed green salad, and whole grain toast

Snack: Greek yogurt with sliced apple

Dinner: Grilled fish, quinoa (GI: 53, GL: 10), and roasted vegetables

Mastering GI and GL empowers readers to take concrete steps toward stable blood sugar and long-term health. Like a compass, these tools guide daily choices, supporting the book's central message: informed, consistent action is the key to reversing type 2 diabetes and reclaiming well-being.

Bibliography

Ahmed, Fatema, et al. "Dietary Patterns and Type 2 Diabetes Risk in Asian Populations: A Systematic Review." *Nutrients* 13, no. 11 (2021): 4134. https://doi.org/10.3390/nu13114134.

American Diabetes Association. "Standards of Medical Care in Diabetes—2024." *Diabetes Care* 47, no. Supplement 1 (2024): S1–S320. https://doi.org/10.2337/dc24-Sint.

Barnard, Neal D., et al. "A Low-Fat Vegan Diet Improves Glycemic Control and Cardiovascular Risk Factors in a Randomized Clinical Trial in Individuals with Type 2 Diabetes." *Diabetes Care* 29, no. 8 (2006): 1777–83.

Basu, Sanjay, et al. "Dietary Patterns and Type 2 Diabetes: A Systematic Literature Review and Meta-Analysis of Prospective Studies." *European Journal of Epidemiology* 29, no. 5 (2014): 231–45.

Boden, G. "Obesity, Insulin Resistance and Free Fatty Acids." *Current Opinion in Endocrinology, Diabetes and Obesity* 18, no. 2 (2011): 139–43.

Centers for Disease Control and Prevention. "National Diabetes Statistics Report, 2022."

https://www.cdc.gov/diabetes/data/statistics-report/index.html.

Chatterjee, Sudesna, et al. "Type 2 Diabetes Control and Complications in Rural India: A 10-Year Follow-Up Study." *Diabetologia* 63, no. 1 (2020): 190–201.

DeFronzo, Ralph A., et al. "Pathogenesis of Type 2 Diabetes Mellitus." *Medical Clinics of North America* 95, no. 2 (2011): 327–48.

Diabetes Prevention Program Research Group. "Reduction in the Incidence of Type 2 Diabetes with Lifestyle Intervention or Metformin." *New England Journal of Medicine* 346, no. 6 (2002): 393–403.

Evert, Alison B., et al. "Nutrition Therapy for Adults with Diabetes or Prediabetes: A Consensus Report." *Diabetes Care* 42, no. 5 (2019): 731–54.

Foster, Gary D., et al. "Weight and Metabolic Outcomes after 2 Years on a Low-Carbohydrate versus Low-Fat Diet." *Annals of Internal Medicine* 153, no. 3 (2010): 147–57.

Fung, Jason, and Jimmy Moore. *The Diabetes Code: Prevent and Reverse Type 2 Diabetes Naturally.* Vancouver: Greystone Books, 2018.

Gregg, Edward W., et al. "Sustainability of Intensive Lifestyle Intervention in Type 2 Diabetes." *JAMA* 316, no. 7 (2016): 701–2.

Hallberg, Sarah J., et al. "Effectiveness and Safety of a Novel Care Model for the Management of Type 2 Diabetes at One Year: An Open-Label, Non-Randomized, Controlled Study." *Diabetes Therapy* 9, no. 2 (2018): 583–612.

Hu, Frank B. *Obesity Epidemiology.* Oxford: Oxford University Press, 2008.

International Diabetes Federation. "IDF Diabetes Atlas, 10th Edition." Brussels: IDF, 2021. https://diabetesatlas.org/.

Joslin, Elliott P. "Correspondence with W.B. Castle, 1936." Joslin Diabetes Center Archives, Boston, MA.

Lean, Michael E.J., et al. "Primary Care-Led Weight Management for Remission of Type 2 Diabetes (DiRECT): An Open-Label, Cluster-Randomised Trial." *Lancet* 391, no. 10120 (2018): 541–51.

Levin, Simon M. "Plant-Based Diets and Diabetes: A Review." *Current Diabetes Reports* 19, no. 10 (2019): 101.

Li, Guojun, et al. "The Long-Term Effect of Lifestyle Interventions to Prevent Diabetes in the China Da Qing Diabetes Prevention Study: A 20-Year Follow-Up Study." *Lancet* 371, no. 9626 (2008): 1783–89.

Look AHEAD Research Group. "Long-term Effects of a Lifestyle Intervention on Weight and Cardiovascular Risk Factors in Individuals with Type 2 Diabetes Mellitus: Four-Year Results of the Look AHEAD Trial." *Archives of Internal Medicine* 170, no. 17 (2010): 1566–75.

Ludwig, David S., and Cara B. Ebbeling. "The Carbohydrate-Insulin Model of Obesity: Beyond 'Calories In, Calories Out'." *JAMA Internal Medicine* 178, no. 8 (2018): 1098–1103.

Mann, Jim I., and Trish D. R. Jenkins. "Glycemic Index and Glycemic Load for Diabetes Management." *British Journal of Nutrition* 119, no. 1 (2018): 43–50.

NHS. "Type 2 Diabetes – Overview." National Health Service, 2023. https://www.nhs.uk/conditions/type-2-diabetes/.

Pan, Xiaoren, et al. "Effects of Diet and Exercise in Preventing NIDDM in People with Impaired Glucose Tolerance: The Da Qing IGT and Diabetes Study." *Diabetes Care* 20, no. 4 (1997): 537–44.

Petrie, John R., et al. "Management of Type 2 Diabetes: A Consensus Statement by the American Diabetes Association and the European Association for the Study of Diabetes." *Diabetologia* 65, no. 12 (2022): 1925–66.

Polonsky, William H., and Richard R. Rubin. "Psychosocial Factors in Diabetes Management." *Diabetes Care* 25, no. 1 (2002): 267–71.

Robertson, Mary D., et al. "Insulin-Sensitizing Effects of Dietary Resistant Starch and Effects on Skeletal Muscle and Adipose Tissue Metabolism." *American Journal of Clinical Nutrition* 82, no. 3 (2005): 559–67.

Shai, Iris, et al. "Weight Loss with a Low-Carbohydrate, Mediterranean, or Low-Fat Diet." *New England Journal of Medicine* 359, no. 3 (2008): 229–41.

Taylor, Roy. "Type 2 Diabetes: Etiology and Reversibility." *Diabetes Care* 36, no. 4 (2013): 1047–55.

Tuomilehto, Jaakko, et al. "Prevention of Type 2 Diabetes Mellitus by Changes in Lifestyle among Subjects with Impaired Glucose Tolerance." *New England Journal of Medicine* 344, no. 18 (2001): 1343–50.

World Health Organization. "Global Report on Diabetes." Geneva: WHO, 2016. https://www.who.int/publications/i/item/9789241565257.

Annotations Recap:

Barnard et al. (2006): Plant-based diet efficacy

Chatterjee et al. (2020): Rural India/global perspective

Evert et al. (2019): Nutrition therapy guidelines

Fung and Moore (2018): Practical diabetes reversal guide

Joslin (1936): Historical/primary source

Lean et al. (2018): DiRECT remission trial

Mann and Jenkins (2018): Glycemic index/load science

Taylor (2013): Diabetes reversibility research

World Health Organization (2016): Global/epidemiological context

This bibliography provides a robust foundation of scientific, clinical, and historical resources to support the narrative and evidence base of a comprehensive book on reversing type 2 diabetes through practical, sustainable strategies.

Epilogue: A New Chapter in the Story of Health

The Journey Revisited

As we reach the final pages of this book, it's natural to pause and reflect on the journey we've taken together, a journey that has woven together science, personal stories, and practical strategies for reclaiming health from type 2 diabetes. What began, for many, as a diagnosis cloaked in uncertainty and fear has, through knowledge and action, become a story of empowerment and hope.

Type 2 diabetes, once considered a lifelong, progressively worsening condition, now stands at the threshold of a paradigm shift. The evidence is clear, the tools are at hand, and the stories of those who have reversed or controlled their diabetes are no longer rare exceptions but growing testaments to what is possible.

Synthesizing the Science and the Stories

Throughout this book, we have explored the mechanisms of type 2 diabetes, the role of diet and exercise, the science of the glycemic index, the promise of plant-based nutrition, and the importance of stress management, sleep, and social support. Each chapter has contributed a vital piece to the puzzle, forming a comprehensive, actionable framework for change.

Key Insights

Type 2 diabetes is largely preventable and, for many, reversible. The body has an incredible capacity to heal when given the right conditions—especially in the early stages of diabetes.

Diet is foundational. Understanding the glycemic index/glycemic load and prioritizing whole, unprocessed foods can dramatically improve blood sugar control.

Movement matters. Regular physical activity sensitizes the body to insulin and supports overall metabolic health.

Mindset and environment are crucial. Stress reduction, adequate sleep, and supportive relationships amplify the benefits of dietary and activity changes.

Cultural context shapes outcomes. Adapting strategies to fit individual backgrounds, values, and resources increases the likelihood of lasting success.

These insights are not just theoretical—they are lived realities for countless people who have reclaimed their health, often against formidable odds. Their stories are proof that change is possible, regardless of background, age, or circumstance.

Societal Implications: A Call for Transformation

The implications of reversing type 2 diabetes extend far beyond individual well-being. At a broader level, the lessons learned have the potential to transform families, communities, and even nations.

The Economic and Social Burden

Globally, type 2 diabetes imposes a staggering burden—measured not only in medical costs but in lost productivity, diminished quality of life, and premature death. In many countries, diabetes care consumes a significant portion of healthcare budgets, diverting resources from other pressing needs.

By empowering people to prevent and reverse type 2 diabetes, we can reduce this burden, improve economic resilience, and enhance social cohesion. Every person who regains their health becomes an advocate, a role model, and a catalyst for change in their circle of influence.

Equity and Accessibility

It is essential, however, to recognize that not everyone enjoys equal access to healthy foods, safe spaces for exercise, or supportive healthcare systems. Addressing the root causes of health disparities—such as poverty, food deserts, and lack of education—must be part of any comprehensive strategy.

Community gardens in urban neighborhoods, culturally tailored nutrition education programs, and affordable access to healthcare are just a few examples of how societies can work together to create environments where healthy choices are truly accessible to all.

The Power of Collective Action

History has shown that major health challenges—like polio, HIV/AIDS, or smallpox—have been overcome not only by scientific breakthroughs but by collective will and cooperation. The same spirit is required now to turn the tide against type 2 diabetes.

This means moving beyond blame and stigma, and instead fostering empathy, support, and empowerment. It means advocating for policies that prioritize public health, food justice, and environmental sustainability. And it means recognizing that each of us has a role to play—in our families, workplaces, and communities.

Looking Forward: The Future of Diabetes Reversal

As we look to the future, the momentum for diabetes reversal continues to build. New research, technological innovations, and community-led initiatives are expanding the possibilities for prevention and recovery.

Emerging Technologies and Personalized Medicine

Digital health platforms, wearable devices, and continuous glucose monitors now make it easier than ever to track progress, receive personalized feedback, and stay motivated. Advances in genomics and precision nutrition promise to further tailor recommendations to individual needs, optimizing outcomes and minimizing guesswork.

The Rise of Holistic, Integrative Care

Healthcare systems are increasingly recognizing the value of integrative approaches—combining medical care with nutrition counseling, exercise therapy, psychological support, and peer mentoring. This shift reflects a growing understanding that health is not merely the absence of disease, but a dynamic state of physical, emotional, and social well-being.

Global Movements and Grassroots Leadership

Around the world, grassroots movements are reclaiming food sovereignty, promoting indigenous foodways, and building networks of support for those living with diabetes. Whether it's community kitchens in Brazil, yoga-based programs in India, or indigenous health cooperatives in Australia, these efforts demonstrate the power of local leadership and cultural wisdom.

An Invitation to Write Your Own Story

As you close this book, you stand at the threshold of your own new chapter. The path to lasting health is not always linear, and setbacks may occur. But every step, no matter how small, is an act of courage and self-care.

Remember:

You are not alone. Millions have walked this path, and a global community stands ready to support you.
Every choice counts. Small, consistent actions compound over time to create profound transformation.
Your story matters. By sharing your journey, you inspire others to believe in what is possible.

Be the Change

The reversal of type 2 diabetes is more than a medical achievement—it is a testament to human potential and resilience. It is a story of reclaiming agency, restoring hope, and building a healthier future for all.

Let us honor the lessons of the past, celebrate the successes of the present, and shape a future where type 2 diabetes is no longer a silent epidemic but a challenge we have learned to overcome—together.

Take the first step today. Reflect on your own habits, reach out for support, and commit to positive change. Share your knowledge, advocate for healthier communities, and become a beacon of hope in a world hungry for healing.

The story of reversing type 2 diabetes fast—and for good—is still being written. May your journey be a source of strength, inspiration, and lasting health.

www.ingramcontent.com/pod-product-compliance
Lightning Source LLC
Chambersburg PA
CBHW081413270326
41931CB00015B/3257

9 781960 833112